THREE D__

WEEKS

My fight for a life without alcohol

KEVIN BARNETT

WORDCATCHER publishing

Three Desperate Weeks
My fight for a life without alcohol
Wordcatcher True Stories

Source images supplied by Adobe Stock
Cover design © 2018 David Norrington

British Library Cataloguing in Publication Data.
A catalogue record for this book is available from the British Library.

Published in the United Kingdom by Wordcatcher Publishing Group Ltd www.wordcatcher.com
Tel: 02921 888321
Facebook.com/WordcatcherPublishing

First Edition: 2018
Print edition ISBN: 9781789420326
Ebook edition ISBN: 9781789420333

Category: Autobiography / Biography / True Stories and Real Lives

CONTENTS

DEDICATION AND ACKNOWLEDGEMENTS

This work is dedicated to:

My beloved wife Jan, because of whom, I am, without any doubt, the luckiest man alive.

To the staff of:

The South Western Ambulance Service NHS Foundation Trust for the life-saving rapid response, and the care of both teams caring for me during the journeys to the Royal Cornwall Hospital, Treliske, Truro and Derriford Hospital, Plymouth.

The Royal Cornwall Hospitals NHS Trust: The Royal Cornwall Hospital, Treliske, Truro, for saving my life in Accident and Emergency and stabilising my condition in Intensive Care sufficiently for me to receive my TIPSS procedure. The TIPSS procedure will be explained in Chapter Eight of the story.

Plymouth Hospitals NHS Trust: Derriford Hospital, Plymouth, Devon for their expertise in performing the TIPSS procedure and the care afforded to me by the wonderful staff of the Intensive Care Unit and the Marlborough Ward.

I wish that I could individually name all those staff who worked together to save my life. Their care started my never-ending recovery from alcohol and enabled me to get on with my life with a markedly changed perspective. Unfortunately, I am not in a position to do this. However, I will never forget them, their skill, and above all, compassion.

Blood donors everywhere, for the selfless act of giving blood and blood products. You save the lives of people you never even meet. It may sound hackneyed, but I believe blood (and organ) donation to be an act of unconditional human compassion because of this.

I gratefully acknowledge: my sister-in-law, Kathryn Horler-Clee; my wife's cousin, Adrian Dolecki; and his partner, Helen Latham, for their love and support to Jan, and myself, as well as reminding me that I do still have family.

Peter and Eiryl Wells for literally going the extra mile, visiting me at Derriford Hospital in Devon, and reminding me of what real friends are all about.

Christine Davies, Carol Smith and Margaret Cresci for their friendship and always being there for us.

PROLOGUE

The story told here happened to my wife and I in late 2015. For us it was a true horror story. It frightened us to our very cores, somewhere even the scariest of fictional horror never gets close to.

Personally, I have no doubt that my experiences are common to many. I have fought for many years, am still fighting, and will always have to fight, the terrible twin demons of depression and alcoholism.

I am not ashamed of my alcoholism, and I do not consider it, or suffering from depression, to be a weakness. They are illnesses. They are also integral parts of me and contribute, along with the many other contradictions I possess as a complex human being, to make the sum of the whole of who I am.

The following is a very brief, illuminating, paraphrased, exchange between the actor, the late Richard Burton CBE, and Michael Parkinson during an interview for the latter's BBC television chat show in 1974.

> *Michael Parkinson: "...if you don't commit suicide, how do you kill yourself?"*
> *Richard Burton: "...you can drink yourself to death, which is really rather pleasant."*

I can't imagine how incredibly difficult it must have been for Richard Burton, arguably the finest actor of his generation, unbelievably famous for that in itself and his two marriages to Elizabeth Taylor, not to mention all-round man's man; to be so honest in talking about his own state of mind and alcoholism, (on television too) some forty-four years ago.

You could be forgiven for thinking from Burton's quote that he is being incredibly flippant about the whole business of drinking and it being a method of achieving one's own death. However, if you are ever lucky enough to watch the whole of this interview (or watch it again if you are old enough to have seen it the first time round) I hope you would appreciate that being flippant he is not. He was engaged in a never-ending fight with his demons and what other way was there forty-four years ago but to put the heroic face on – at least in public. It is unfortunate that in the years which have passed since the Parkinson interview, that men and women very often still have to present their drinking as mock-heroic, to make a joke about it, in a society that generally remains reluctant to discuss mental illness and alcoholism openly, as the third decade of the 21st century approaches.

Not that I do, would, or could, compare myself in any way to the great actor and my fellow Welshman; but the point is that what happened to him and me, with regard to depression and alcoholism, could happen to anyone. Both depression and alcoholism are dreadful diseases. They afflict indiscriminately in a society which still holds undue prejudice towards, and stigmatises those who are, so afflicted.

A great deal of work must be done by all who have it within their power to contribute to tackling these diseases, and the social consequences of them. That includes people like me, who have not been so unlucky as to have been permanently robbed by depression and alcoholism of their capacity to contribute to the debate, and hopefully to finding the way forward for treatment and care.

I do not have a plan for how this could or should be done. I have neither the kind nor level of resources necessary to combat these diseases strategically within our communities. I am, after all, only one person who has terrible first-hand experience of them, from which I have decided to write an honest, at times nakedly so, account of my own experiences at the mercies of depression and alcoholism. Indeed, you could be forgiven for thinking at times, 'too much information!' However, I have included details of everyday life, especially whilst I was convalescing on Marlborough Ward that will hopefully convey how my drinking took away my dignity. I was reduced from a highly-functioning, independent and confident man, to a needy, crying wreck, dependent upon strangers, albeit caring ones, to help with basic bodily functions. If you have, or think you have, a problem with alcohol addiction, seek help before it takes your dignity.

Despite the introduction of the Health and Social Care Act 2012, creating the legal responsibility for the NHS to deliver 'parity of esteem' between treating physical and mental health, there still remains a great deal of work to be done to eradicate the stigmas in our society which have, for some reason, become attached, limpet-like, to mental illness and the conditions associated with it, such as alcoholism.

And what of alcoholics? Look at those around you, and then yourself if you drink. You, and any one, or more, of your friends or family could be (or are quite likely to be if 'safe drinking' guidelines are any sort of measure to be trusted) 'drinking too much', be a 'binge' or 'problem drinker', or even a 'high functioning alcoholic' like I was for many years, before it all got too much for me and the frail bodily shell of my humanity. People don't have to conform to stereotypes, such as lying in gutters, clutching crumpled brown paper bags containing empty bottles of 'Emva Cream', soaked and covered in their own piss, shit and vomit, to qualify as alcoholics, or some lesser version on the boozers' continuum thereof.

If you drink alcohol, but fail to respect it, you will fit in to one of the above codifications – 'binge drinker' is the most likely one. It's so *easy* to join that club. Call it 'entry level' into the drinker's club, if you like. The thing is, though, that it is also *frighteningly* easy for any drinker to upgrade their membership from there. I paid my dues regularly and keenly, eager to move my way up to the very top echelons of the club. I did it. I reached the dizzying heights of seniority only to find out it was the longest, hardest sobering of falls back to the reality of solid ground.

I was extremely lucky to be given the chance to fight another day. I was given what would be described in today's parlance, 'binary choices': i) to drink or not to drink, ii) to live or to die, and within those two choices the following dichotomy of death or survival: iii) to live fast and die fast, or iv) to live fast and die agonizingly slowly, v) to live in abstinence and hope for the best. I chose option v). You'll get to understand what I mean by "hope for the best" in the Epilogue of this story. "Fight", by the way, is neither too big nor dramatic a verb to use here. For fight is what all depressives have to do to see the light, if they still want to, and recovering alcoholics must do so every single day of their lives to stay sober and, in many cases like mine, even alive.

Sadly, there is no cure for alcoholism, or the cirrhosis of the liver I now have, and speaking as someone not clinically qualified but as a sufferer who has spent, and continues to spend, too much time in the dark corners of despair, I don't personally believe that there is necessarily one for depression either. I am an alcoholic and always will be. At best I will always be a recovering alcoholic. My mental illness is still a part of me, and, I suppose, it will always be lurking somewhere in the background, waiting for an opportunity, a chink to appear in the defences I have set up, to have a go at me once again. Indeed, during the time it has taken me to write this short work, I have suffered several periods of blackness.

Before going any further, I must acknowledge that I was given the chance to fight another day by people who did not judge me as being a hopeless drunk, or someone who should simply "pull himself together"; but rather showed me love, friendship, support and respect, despite everything I, and my illnesses, put them through. I was extremely lucky in this respect also, and I thank all of them here and now.

PART ONE

'SHE'
ALMOST KILLS ME…

ONE

INTRODUCING MY CAUTIONARY TALE

Let me hold up my thankfully now steady hands and say that I truly did love alcohol. Moreover, despite everything that unfolds in the telling of my brief cautionary tale, I still do.

One probably shouldn't humanise anything that isn't human. Doing so is not a reflection of reality and is, therefore, escapism – in this case unhealthily so. Alcohol is very definitely not human. Wow! Bet you didn't realise that, did you? But the obvious needs to be said here because alcohol can, and so very often does, take almost all that is human away from a person. Despite this, I have referred to alcohol as my 'mistress', my 'friend with benefits', my 'tart', my 'little Russian girl', my 'pacifier', (both physical and emotional), the 'girl whose easy time I pay for', or simply, and most predominantly, just 'she' or 'her'.

I felt that to refer to alcohol as merely 'alcohol' didn't acknowledge its lofty position in the hierarchy of the significant relationships in my life. So, for the purposes of this story, I'd been having dark times, when I could not, or most likely chose not, to see the inherent dangers of an indulgent relationship with alcohol, I gave it these tempting and alluring, if somewhat stereotypically shallow, even celluloid-like, fantasy female roles and attributes.

When I think about it now with, for the time being anyway (for there are no guarantees of forever sobriety amongst the alcoholics' fraternity), a clear head; there are parallels that can quite reasonably be drawn between the ferocious intensity of the damaging relationship between alcohol and the alcoholic and that of the corrosive, unfulfilled love of a man who returns, time and again, to have his heart broken by the woman who is the object of his unrequited desire, love and affection.

Of course, alcohol doesn't know this and the poor analogous 'woman' will often be, if not oblivious to what is going on, simply at a loss for coping with the persistency of unwanted attention.

This is a traditional allegory then. It is a rehashed old moral story, where the protagonist, in this case a reasonably intelligent man (me, believe it or not), who did not possess the strength to follow the right path, fell hopelessly under the spell of a beautiful, but dangerous, friend with benefits, who could not reciprocate his feelings. More importantly, 'she' could not help him in his hours of need, when he turned to her for release from the darkness of his everyday existence. She was a mistress, whose corrupting nature took control of him, so overwhelmingly, that he came as close as was possible to being forever subjugated by her... in death.

To begin with, 'she' was my friend with benefits. She was one to enjoy with guaranteed satisfaction, but without any commitment on my part. Indeed, in what now seems like a different life, I wouldn't see or hear from her for weeks and months on end. I simply didn't need to drink the poisoned *eau de vie* she offered me. I was, at the beginning of it all, easily satisfied without excess of her.

If only it could have stayed that way. Just the occasional intimate encounter. But then I fell insanely in love with her, this intoxicatingly bewitching mistress, whom I had to have with me constantly. Over time, I lost my independence as a man and my mind and body could not function without her.

Rather like a brothel menu, sometimes my mistress would be a gutter slut white cider, which had never even seen an apple, sometimes she was an elegant and refined courtesan in the form of an expensive Krug champagne; and at all other times, everything in between. I consumed her in whatever way I could afford, and the more variety she offered me, the more exciting she became. This was perverse, as I was able to have her at any time the excitement should have diminished. Except, of course, ultimately, I did not see when the excitement had given way to dependency.

She was my *eau de vie*.

But, as is the case with many a relationship, I

became somewhat complacent with her presence, and the enjoyment she gave me. So not long ago, she threw me a curveball in order to regain my attention. In hindsight, I should not have considered her actions to be a nasty surprise or rebuke. I knew that I wasn't respecting her, and she was merely pointing out my lack of manners.

Our relationship has not ended, but rather it has transformed into an infinite struggle to keep her at arm's length, and me out of her intimate, vice-like, deadly clutches, where we would inevitably consume each other in a conflagration which she would walk away from, leaving me for dead this time.

The relentless longing, and gnawing away at one's centre of reasoning, to be reconciled with her, never goes away. Only another recovering alcoholic can fully appreciate the meaning of that statement. Oh, to taste her once more! To have that slow burn ignite within me as I ingest her, or have her quench, ice-cold, a summer thirst would be such a pleasant assault on my celibate senses. But one knows that to resume that intimacy would, with absolutely no doubt, result in an encounter so intense that the shock of it would be lethal, either acutely or chronically (but still in the relatively short term). Having said all that, I have to confess to still thinking sometimes, what a perverse blessing it would be, to slip without pain into that dark, velvety, comfortable and infinite oblivion.

TWO

THE DREADFUL CARNAGE OF THE WEE-SMALL HOURS

In the early hours of 5th November 2015, 'she' caused me to be admitted to hospital as an emergency, and thereafter to spend, what turned out to be a surreal three weeks of experiences good and bad, light (only with hindsight) and nightmarishly dark.

I was getting ready to go to bed at around 2am. I was in the bathroom of our holiday cottage, 'straining the greens', as they say. Suddenly, without any warning in the form of nausea or pain, a substantial volume of dark red liquid shot out of my mouth, without any effort at all, ending up all over the toilet and the floor in front of me. The bath adjacent to the toilet accumulated about an inch of this sticky purple, claret coloured looking liquid in the tap end.

I tried to kid myself by thinking that it was just red wine (mixed with God knows what else and in what quantity) coming back up, but I knew it wasn't really. This regurgitate was lumpy, and those lumps were jelly-like, and there was no partly digested food in it. It was thick and tacky. Moreover, it had that unmistakable iron taste of blood. I later found out that it was this colour and consistency because it wasn't fresh blood and I had been bleeding internally for some time, hence its partial coagulation. This is what it was like to start off with anyway, for the subsequent episodes of blood-vomiting would be bright red and of a thinner consistency because it was fresh.

I pulled myself together as best I could, incredibly managed to clean myself up and the mess around me without waking my wife and went to bed very worried. Idiotically, I tried to convince myself, against the odds, that things would be OK in the morning, provided I didn't vomit again. Oh no, no, no! An hour or so later, due to my age, I was up again to use the bathroom. While relieving myself, I belched, and the red fountain was opened again. Like I hadn't already known it, my inner monologue advised me that I was in serious trouble here.

I sat down on the bloody toilet seat, my heart pounding, and breathing becoming more laboured and feeling less effective, and a third great surge of blood, projected by high pressure, shot forth from my mouth. The bathroom took on the appearance of a scene from an American teenage slasher movie, or the Normandy beaches landings as they were graphically depicted in the film, *Saving Private Ryan*. Blood had hit every corner of the bathroom, and the whole floor was awash with it. I myself was covered in blood from my mouth down. It was running down in rivulets and dripping off me.

There was no hiding this from my wife, and no point in trying, because it was only going to happen again until I had no blood left in me. There was also another necessity to awaken her. I could well succumb just sat there, and she would walk in on me some time later and be shockingly confronted by me not only looking like the central figure in an horrific zombie portrait, but, well...dead, for real.

Believe me, preserving my wife's sanity, (at least in an immediate sense, as I'm sure it was resoundingly tested later) was my overriding concern. I wasn't bothered about being saved. I really wasn't. My depression, upon which I'll expand in the proceeding chapters and in my next book, had it seemed, switched off the human survival instinct in me. It had taken the very desire for life away from me. I just didn't want my wife sleepily walking into the bathroom and being freaked out by the corpse of her dead husband, looking like the character *Beetlejuice* covered in blood, sitting on the toilet, surrounded by a veritable lake of more blood.

I called out for my wife from my bloody throne. It must have been about four or five times before she heard me through her slumber. Added to that, my voice had diminished along with my blood and strength levels. She eventually came in, and after the initial shock of seeing me covered in all that blood, she put in motion what would happen over the next most unusual and life-changing three weeks.

THREE

WHY DO ANYTHING?

The opening of this tale has been penned dark and despondent. This was necessary in order to convey the terrifying, deeply intestinal shock, of vomiting one's life blood away. Vomiting and vomiting my own blood until there was almost none of it left.

Perhaps I should provide some background to the situation in the cottage bathroom, in order for the reader to fill in a few gaps about my life as it was at the time, and had been, on and off, for at least the two or three decades before, by way of explaining why this was happening to me.

"It was the depression what did it, Guv." The causes of my depression, as I deduced them to be some time ago, and the subsequent impact that my depression was having upon my life, and on those around me, led inevitably to what happened during the early hours of 5th November 2015.

I did think about expanding upon my depression, including its causes and dimensions, in this story. However, when I got to the end of the first draft, and began to revisit it for refining purposes, I made up my mind that I would not.

In order for anyone else to fully appreciate the role that depression had played in my circumstances, and therefore its influence on my drinking, I considered that it was more appropriate, even necessary, to write about my depression in its own right. Therefore, the story of my depression will be explored in a separate work reflecting on the twenty-five years or so leading up to the three desperate weeks in November 2015.

Anyway, I'd been having a particularly bad and lingering bout of depression for at least the five years leading up to November 2015. During this time, for the most part I had been a 'functioning' alcoholic. I was just about holding down a responsible job, trying outwardly to appear as 'normal' as possible. In private, though, I was doing weird things such as eating bowls of Smash (instant mashed potato) mixed with vast amounts of butter and Heinz (it had to be Heinz) salad cream, washed down with a bottle of red, while sat in bed watching the morning news before going to work. I was *always* drinking. I would drink before, during and after work; and all times over the weekends...

I had got to the stage where I would get out of bed in the morning, sometimes I would shower, sometimes I wouldn't bother. However, the latter was becoming the norm. I wouldn't bother to shower because it was no longer important to me, and in order to maximise the amount of time I would have before going in to work for drinking purposes. My wife visited her gym three days of the week, which meant her leaving the house at about 6am in the morning, spending an hour in the gym, before going straight to work from there. If it was one of those days, I would get up as soon as I heard her close the front door behind her. Checking she had left the house, and had pulled away in her car from the drive, without further ado, I would start drinking, straight from the bottle, either lying in bed, or move the considerable distance, sloth-like, to the living room and my faithful old armchair in front of the television overlooking our balcony with a view of the street below. This was a particularly good vantage point to keep a close eye, just in case my wife returned home for some reason rather than go straight to work from the gym. There was the odd occasion when she did do this and having spied her car pulling up, I would 'close everything down', by hiding my bottle and going into the bathroom to clean my teeth as if I was just getting up.

I would get through a bottle of wine usually before leaving for work, although there were some occasions when I over did the pre-work drink to the extent that I knew I could not have hidden my inebriation from colleagues, let alone be sufficiently co-ordinated to drive the ten or so miles to the office. I had probably mixed the wine with something stronger, such as vodka, some of my wife's gin or even brandy – all in the same glass together. I had some very interesting pre-work cocktails. There were, what I would call, 'legitimate' bottles of spirits (those bought by my wife, or my wife and I, for holidays, left over from Christmas and so on) in the house that had been surreptitiously 'replaced' by me dozens of times over. On the occasions I thought it best not to go into work, I would hastily contact the office on some pretext for needing to take a day's leave. Needless to say, I would spend the remainder of such days taking my state of drunkenness to greater heights, or perhaps lower depths would be a more appropriate description of the direction of travel.

Sometimes, on the drive to work, I would stop at the garage or supermarket to purchase a bottle of red wine and sometimes one of vodka. I kept an empty 500ml 'Ribena Light' (I was at least a calorie controlled drunk) bottle in my car. Sitting in the car park of the garage or supermarket, I would fill this plastic bottle with red wine, or red wine mixed with vodka. Visually, anyone, except perhaps for the likes of me, would be hard pressed to tell the difference between it and the red herring soft drink. I would then proceed to drink this in the car on my way to the office, refilling the bottle in the office car park before entering the building. Sat at my desk, I would drink from it all day just to keep me on an even keel and to keep the pain of everyday reality at bay. Lunchtimes I would go out to a local shop and buy more red wine so that I could keep filling my Ribena Light bottle during the afternoon.

I would even take a full one of my booze-filled Ribena Light bottles into meetings with me and sit there slurping away, while the others drank water, tea or coffee – or at least I assume that's what they were all drinking, but one never really knows, does one? To ensure that my breath never gave me away, I always had an abundance of mints or chewing gum with me. I was a perpetual chewer. I even came up with the idea of disguising my boozy breath with clove oil. Being particularly pungent, I was sure that this would mask anything I drank. The smell of the clove oil in its own right drew attention to me, of course, but all I had to say was that I had a toothache. Actually, that wasn't so very far from the truth a lot of the time, as my teeth have suffered probably every bit as much as my liver has from the effects of my alcoholism. Nibbling on raw cloves of garlic was another reliable method of throwing people off the scent of the booze on my breath. This was, though, less socially acceptable, so I used this ploy at home more than at work. I would continue to drink during the drive home and call in to the local garage store, or wherever, for supplies for the night. I had overcome the drinker's nightmare of running out of booze or the problem of work getting in the way of drinking. Drinking was truly 24/7 for me. It was the proudest achievement of that period of my life...

However, while describing myself as a functioning alcoholic, I also missed a great deal of work during this time. As I sat at home alone, drinking heavily and constantly ruminating over how 'sad' my life was, I became oblivious to all that was good about it.

Another way of looking at it was that the beauty of life all around me, intense and vibrant with brightness, colour, smell and sound as it was, became too much to bear. It jarred and jangled on my senses and nerves. Then there came a time when I couldn't appreciate any of this anyway, as I became totally encapsulated by what seemed an impenetrable bubble of greyness.

I just didn't care about anything anymore – myself, least of all. The day was spent drinking, drinking some more, drinking a lot more; and then falling asleep, waking up to find that 'she' had run out on me. All my bottles were drained. Sometimes when I was off work my only exercise of body and mind during a typical day was the how and when of the next drink.

I drove my car in this state to a shop to buy more alcohol from shop assistants who judged me and made, just about audible, comments behind my back such as, "I know, and it's only half past eight...", as I paid and scurried away, dishevelled and smelly, to my potentially lethal four wheeled weapon.

This happened every day, several times a day, for months on end. I ended up running out of money, having gone on half and then zero salary. I raided the holiday savings fund for the small change, and our dog Gracie's little fired clay piggy bank, which my niece (a friend's daughter) had made in school for her, containing merely pennies, just in order to make up sufficient monies to buy a bottle of my gutter slut's booze.

I dreaded the payment transactions. First dread, as I approached the shop: would it be the same person who had served me at the same time yesterday morning? There was one long, grey-haired North Walian woman who, it seemed to me, always took the breakfast shift in the Tesco Express store on the main road.

Don't forget, that by the time I was making my first purchase of the day, all liquid of course, I was already a few sheets to the wind. It was a continuous process, you see, with almost always a bottle of something inside me to tide me over until the licensing laws would permit the local shops to sell me more alcohol.

I would pull up outside the little Tesco, in my Peripatetic Potential Killing machine. In fact, I was, what might be chillingly described as, 'road licenced to kill'. This terrible 007 play on words isn't meant to be clever or funny. I use it because it is somewhat apt to describe the despicable act that I was committing in getting into my car, drunk. I could well have killed or maimed indiscriminately. We were all very lucky that I never did.

I would go into the shop, dishevelled, for the first of my purchases that day. I was convinced that the North Walian woman was judging me. Indeed, I still believe that she was even now that I am sober. For all the looking down her nose at me, however, and despite my obvious physical state, she and no other member of staff in that shop, or any of the others I rocked up to several times a day, every day of the week, ever refused to sell me alcohol.

The other part of what I shall call 'transaction dread' was the shaking of my hands. My hands shook for a couple of reasons. The first reason was the more obvious one – delirium tremens. The second was that I was perpetually nervous and embarrassed about continually purchasing alcohol from the same people every day, several times a day, so much so that my hands shook quite violently. Trying to hit the correct buttons on the credit card machine became a new skill to be mastered. It was almost like what is called, 'Kentucky Windage', when shooting; only in this case making allowances for where the fingers were coming from, and their angle of impact upon the numbered keys of the pad, rather than a bullet or shot hitting a moving target. I failed very regularly to hit the required four digits at the first attempt, which despite being drunk, caused intense embarrassment, and made the situation even worse.

However, the worst was having to pay for my liquor with loose change – especially when I had to make the payment up from the small coins in the holiday savings jar or the dog's piggy bank. This was so humiliating, more so when there was the added pressure of other customers waiting to be served behind me. Imagine counting small change when you are drunk, with insanely shaky hands and fingers that have the stability of an epileptic poltergeist.

I would usually purchase just two bottles of wine on the morning visit to the shops. There was a time when I tried to convince myself that in doing so I could limit the amount I would drink to that for the day. No chance! These would last until about 10:30am which necessitated a further visit to the shops, driving now even more under the influence. Don't forget either that I wouldn't have eaten anything at this point. I'd go straight back home, with another couple of bottles, bought from a different shop to stop the assistants thinking I was a drunk. What a 'plonker', as I returned to the same shops every day anyway. Miraculously, having made it to the shops and back without incident, I would get back into my chair in front of the television and carry on drinking. I didn't use a glass. I drank straight from the bottle.

The effects of the first two bottles of wine of the morning slightly slowed down my consumption of the second two bottles. By mid-afternoon, I would normally be dozing, just on the edge of consciousness, still able to hear the television. When I became fully awake, I would immediately pick up my bottle, if I had had presence of mind to put it down and carry on necking away at it. Late afternoon would arrive. Four bottles down my throat. My wife would usually be home in half an hour. There would be just enough time to visit the garage now to get something else to tide me over for the evening and very early morning the next day before the 8:30am booze run. Who needed Dover to Calais?

The volume of booze I was getting through would have been truly staggering and frightening for anyone observing me in my self-destruct mode. If I could have been sober for long enough and looked at myself drinking with focused purpose of mind, even I would have been scared. But that didn't happen. I just wanted more and more and more of her.

Indeed, when something new came out by a booze producer I respected or liked, I had to try it to see about adding it to my brothel menu of booze. For instance, I remember when Smirnoff brought out their special edition of apple flavoured vodka. I got some, "for a change" you understand. At first, I liked it. It was quite pleasant. The local Co-op store had an opening special offer on it, as did others. Two bottles for £20. By the time I had finished off the second bottle one afternoon, I threw it all back up and decided that I didn't like it anymore. That didn't stop me buying two more bottles of it again the following day for as long as it was on offer.

I didn't eat, I didn't shower; sometimes for a whole week at a time. I didn't do anything but drink, smell and exist. So, what? Who cared?

* * *

I never told anyone that there had been several times during this five-year period of particularly severe depression (if that is indeed how long it was in my poor addled brain's recollection), that I had contemplated taking my own life, planned how I would go about it, and one night attempted to go through with it.

First, I thought about hanging myself from the top of the stairs. Our home was a three-storey property in the 'townhouse' style, the top and final flight of stairs having a good length of drop from where, once over the bannister, there would be no returning. Then I thought what about drugs? An overdose. Less painful and messy. Indeed, a much better option for a coward like me. I was, of course, extremely naïve. I have subsequently learnt that overdoses of painkilling drugs can lead to a distressing death, as the liver slowly dies within the body while the victim is 'acutely aware', I'll put it that way, of it happening.

One night, I went to bed early, about 8pm, and started the process of putting an end to myself, and out of the collective misery, as I saw it, of those who were having to put up with me. I had quite a large number of co-dydramol 30/500's leftover from a prescription I had been given in the A&E Department of my local hospital a year or two before. I had been prescribed them for an injury I had sustained to my left foot while walking the South

West Coast Path on holiday. Upon my return home, and a visit to A&E, it was discovered that I had torn ligaments and a severe sprain, resulting in considerable pain. Hence the large number of strong painkillers being in my possession.

I started to take these leftover drugs. These drugs contained both codeine and paracetamol. I knew that the codeine in the tablets would help to relax me, but it would be the paracetamol that would provide the life-ending poison. I took a handful of these tablets in one go. I didn't know how many it would be necessary to take in order to bring about my fatal poisoning. However, I was counting on taking a lot more. In any event, the paracetamol wouldn't be the only poison in my system. I simultaneously took a handful of my sertraline 100mg anti-depressants too.

The co-dydramol tablets were soluble in water. However, as a belt and braces job, I dissolved them on this occasion in an extremely large quantity of Mr. Smirnoff's red label tart. I kept my little Russian girl in the corner of my part of the bedroom wardrobe, under some shoes. This contraband hiding place had been 'busted' already several times by my wife, but I continued to use it for brief hiding periods only, a sort of holding area for supplies in transit to more secure concealment locations within the house. On this occasion, of course, my Moscow mistress was in just the right place for me to access her. By dissolving the tablets in hard liquor, she would be placing a final soothing hand upon my troubled brow as I hopefully slipped away. I also swallowed the anti-depressants with her help.

Due to the layout of our townhouse, our bedroom was just across a small half-landing from the living room where my poor wife, oblivious to what I was up to in the bedroom with my Russian doll and 'sweeties', was watching television. All the while that I was doing this, I could hear the normality of the sound of the television in the living room. 'Living' room! And here I was in what was about to become the 'death' room. The irony of that was lost on me at the time, but how cruel it would have been for my wife to have come to bed after the normality of watching television and found me gone or unresponsive on my way to Purgatory.

I was sat on the edge of the bed in semidarkness with just the light of the en-suite bathroom behind providing me with the backlit illumination I required for my activities. My eyes brimmed with tears. I felt so sad. Then the coward in me said "stop!" I put my head on my pillow and quietly soaked it with my tears. As it happens, it didn't take me long to fall asleep that night (a rarity) due to the exhausting enormity of what I had been contemplating in taking my own life; and the nerve-numbing interaction of paracetamol, codeine, sertraline and alcohol that was going on in my blood. Being honest, I'm not sure if this was a cry for help, or a serious attempt at taking my own life.

Either way, it was academic really, as due to the failure of my nerve in completing the attempt, I was still around to drink yet another day...

That is the reason for the title of this chapter. The early hours incident in our holiday cottage had, in effect, presented me with the perfect means for everything being over. I would neither have to plan the how and when, nor implement the means. Moreover, the coward within me would no longer have the power to stop this incident from reaching its fruition in my death.

The saddest part of those early hours of 5th November was cleaning up after the initial regurgitation of blood. My wife was still mercifully asleep, but even so she was but a few feet away from the bathroom door. I didn't want her to know what had happened. In my desperation to clean up, and make like nothing had happened, I was on my hands and knees pathetically scrabbling around in silence, with the screams going off inside my head like rocket fireworks in an insane trajectory, absorbing as much of the blood as I could with the toilet roll.

Once I'd finished cleaning up, I sat on the toilet seat with my head in my hands, the mind inside it racing around, trying desperately to construct some alternative version of the truth that was more palatable than the one I knew was the reality.

FOUR

BLUES AND TWOS TO A&E

By the time the ambulance came to take me God knows where, my body and I (the latter meaning my mind or brain) was in shock from the loss of blood and the sheer terror of seeing it all happen.

My wife had cleaned me up as best she could. I had continued vomiting blood while we were waiting for the ambulance to arrive. At her first sight of it, I don't think that she realised it was blood I was throwing up. I admitted to her that I knew it was. There was no point in trying to say that it was something else now. I cried pitifully "Oh Christ!" every time I brought another, now fresh, bright red blood-load up. I was scared. I must have sounded pathetic.

My colour had taken on a strange, creamy, off-white mother-of-pearl translucency and, of course, I had barely enough strength left to stand up. My mind was whirring. What was going to happen to me?

The wonderful paramedics could not get a trolley or wheelchair into the cottage due to its layout.

They got me to my feet and supported me, one under each arm out of the property and got me into the ambulance. I continued to lose further blood in the ambulance while being whisked away to Treliske Hospital in Truro. This was some forty-five minutes away from where we were staying in the lovely harbour town of Porthleven in the far south of Cornwall.

As we were getting ready to pull away from the cottage, the paramedic ambulance driver told my wife, who was getting into my Land Rover to follow him, not to try to keep up in the event that he had to put the blue lights and siren on, as it could be dangerous for her to do so. He would only do this, he explained, if I took a turn for the worse and he had to hasten our arrival at the hospital. About ten minutes into the journey we got stuck in traffic due to road works. The paramedic ambulance driver had no choice but to light-up and sound-off as my condition could not wait for the traffic to clear. Jan was left behind in the traffic jam obviously thinking that I had taken that turn for the worse...

* * *

Until 'she' put me in this situation, where it was me who required the services of Accident and Emergency, I had been fortunate enough only to have endured the experience vicariously when accompanying someone else who required urgent medical intervention.

I recall on those occasions, that first it was the triage nurse, and then possibly some hours later the person I had been accompanying would be summoned for the first of about half a dozen very brief encounters with a doctor. It had always seemed to me that a significant amount of time was given over to repeated introductions of who we all were, and why we were there. This was because so much time would elapse in between each encounter with the A&E doctor, or doctors, that everyone had forgotten the why's and wherefores.

On this occasion, I was wheeled into A&E at Treliske, pushed on a trolley driven with purpose and speed, straight through the gathered hordes of the injured and 'maybe dying', and parked straightaway in a treatment cubicle. I had bypassed the usual routines of A&E. Thankfully, instead of having to wait what had always seemed to me on those previous occasions, an interminable period to be seen, I was attended to immediately. Such waiting around was not for me. I was haemorrhaging so heavily that to wait could have meant death. That is the way to get seen fast in A&E! Although, this is not a handy tip I wish to pass on to readers. Please don't try this at home, as they say. Some of what was left of my blood was taken and tested for type. I was soon placed on a drip, receiving fluids and sustenance from donated blood and various other fluids, like the starving 'Undead'.

Undead was a good adjective for how I was and

appeared, and the predicament I was in. The thought struck me, for the third time that morning, that I could be close to the time of my death. Indeed, that could have been my last thought. My inner monologue saying, "that could have been my last thought" was also immediate history.

Of course, everything someone thinks, does or says becomes history instantly, but somehow, in these extraordinary circumstances, at least to me they were, this reality seemed to be bright, loud and jarring, like looking directly at the white-hot sun or crunching down hard on an ice cube with sensitive teeth.

Every breath, every blink of my eyes, swallow of my throat, thought in my shocked brain, and terrified gaze into the cubicle curtain in front of me, COULD. BE. IT. I sat there almost too terrified to move, lest I knock my on/off switch to the 'off' position.

At last Jan arrived. Not having been to the hospital before, she had got lost on the drive up and then there was the usual inadequate and overcomplicated parking arrangements to cope with. In the meantime, the A&E staff had been trying their best to fill me back up with blood, but as fast as the units were going in they were coming out again. Apparently, I reached the stage during the next few days (while I was in my induced coma, so I was blissfully unaware) where further blood transfusions / donations could cause other serious complications, including consequences for my liver. This is when things would become incredibly serious, as if they weren't already, because they could not stop the internal bleeding.

In the end it would come down to having an emergency TIPSS procedure (to be explained later) or a liver transplant. If I didn't have the TIPSS procedure, or it didn't work in stopping the bleeding, I would have died as there just aren't livers lying around waiting to be transplanted. I didn't have time to go on the transplant waiting list and wait for one to become available. Unless there was a tragic miracle and someone died so that I could receive their liver ahead of other (definitely more deserving) patients on the waiting list, it was going to be too late.

FIVE

"DO YOU KNOW YOU HAVE A PROBLEM WITH YOUR LIVER?"

Enter the Gastrointestinal and Hepatology Consultant. After introducing himself, he said, "Do you know you have a problem with your liver?"

"No," I lied, with consummate ease.

I bet he thought, *Yeah right you don't!* I could tell immediately from his demeanour that this guy was not going to suffer my foolishness gladly and did not have the time other than to get down to business. He questioned me that no doctor had ever raised the condition of my liver with me before. He examined my abdomen and asked me if I could feel any tenderness or pain anywhere. I answered truthfully this time that I could not. I really could not feel any pain. Now for the forthright bit.

"How much do you drink?"

I'd been anticipating this question.

I'd been asked this question, so many times, over the years by various GPs, because routine blood tests to monitor my liver and kidney function (due to taking prescribed medication to treat hypertension) had often indicated raised Gamma GT levels. Gamma GT (or Gamma-glytamyl transpeptidase to give it its full name), is an enzyme present in the liver, raised levels of which are an indicator of possible liver problems. Mine had nearly always been raised during these tests because I was drinking too much.

I, no doubt like many other people who 'like a bit too much', were 'problem drinkers', 'piss artists' or full-blown 'functioning alcoholics' like me, when asked about how much they drink, substantially downgrade their intake from the sublime to the ridiculous. Instead of making my drinking sound very serious, I made out that it was just very silly, rather like the 'slurps' of the late, and very sadly missed, Keith Floyd.

Believe me, however, I knew that there was nothing funny, or even at best, darkly comedic, about this sad scene of a man still pathetically trying to hide the truth when it was out for all to see.

Not looking the good doctor in the eye, I acted, despite everything that was happening, nonchalant, casual even. I cast my head about the A&E cubicle, and summoned an appropriate number of bottles of an appropriate alcoholic beverage to mind out of the air around us.

"Oh, probably three or four bottles of wine a day, I suppose."

He didn't press me any further on the matter, thankfully, as my poor wife was in attendance. In any event, three or four bottles of wine a day were perfectly adequate for his diagnostic purposes. That much was more than enough to put me in the predicament I was now in. Actually, my drinking far exceeded this volume, and I hadn't just been consuming wine either. I chose catholically from my booze brothel menu of whatever version, and how much of her I could afford.

Anyway, I knew deep down where this conversation was heading. I was still bringing up the red stuff, and the doctor explained what was going to happen. No, I was to have an endoscopy to see what was going on inside me. Oh fuck. That was all I could think. You see, the 'endoscopy' was a procedure I had been secretly terrified of for years – since I was a child, in fact.

Let me explain. In 1967, my father had almost died of a massive intestinal haemorrhage following the perforation of an ulcer, not from alcoholism like his youngest son. He ended up losing half his stomach in what must have been a horrendously scary incident. As soon as I was able to understand what had happened to him, the thought of it, or something like it, happening to me had always been at the back of my mind.

So here it was, happening, sort of. A kind of self-fulfilling prophesy.

I immediately insisted on general anaesthesia. Initially, however, the consultant indicated that this was a luxury I was not going to be afforded due to the risk of complications and, no doubt, the expense. Indeed, I now understand that receiving general anaesthesia for an endoscopy is not usual practice anywhere, unless there are extenuating circumstances of an extreme kind. How was I going to prepare myself for this ordeal? I couldn't even brush my teeth without gagging. I had been that way for some years, no doubt due to the same reasons for which I was drinking and compounded because I was drinking.

I was feeling terrible. My heart was racing, as was my mind. I was in shock. Was this going to be it? I think it was about three or four in the afternoon when they came to take me down to the theatre. The consultant came to the bedside and told me that they had decided I was going to be put out for the procedure. Doubtless it had been determined that my circumstances were of an extreme kind, sufficient to warrant general anaesthesia.

I thanked the consultant, saying something ridiculous like: "You've just made my day, Doctor." I remember him looking at me somewhat incredulously, as I said it. I was to receive a general anaesthetic because I was so acutely ill that the theatre team were hedging their bets as to what was going to happen when I was in there. By knocking me out from the start I would be ready for other, perhaps more open and invasive, interventions should these suddenly become necessary during the endoscopy.

Then, the brakes were released from my bed

and I was on the move, heading for the operating theatre and a date with... I didn't know what altogether. Would I be coming back? Saying goodbye to my wife at that point was probably the saddest thing I had ever had to do thus far in my life. After all, it might not just have been *au revoir.*

It had been entirely different saying goodbye when she had left me in the mornings at home to go to work, and even when I was having suicidal thoughts and making plans; or saying goodnight the evening I went to bed early to take my 'overdose'. Those valedictions hadn't upset me anything like as much.

I didn't show it, but I was crying on the inside as I left her in A&E. She cut a lonely figure as I was wheeled out. God knows how frightened she must have been too. To all intents and purposes, she was all alone. The staff were fantastic, but there was no one familiar at her side. Neither she nor I had control over what was happening, or going to happen, what she might have to cope with. This included, as a very real possibility, even the worst case scenarios.

For all I knew, I might never see her again. It tore me apart until I was anaesthetised, probably about twenty minutes later. That last sentence sounds derisory due to the shortness of time indicated, but it is an accurate one, for I would know nothing of what happened to her, or me, over the next eight days. In fact, I would only come to truly understand what had happened very gradually and little by little over the next three weeks, and counting, as my brain still continues to throw out the odd detail.

I have thought about how sad I felt at this point many times since. I have come to believe that on those occasions when suicide was being contemplated, planned for, and even partially attempted; I was the one who was in control of my immediate fate. I, the coward, could (and did) stop myself from completing the act. Now, I wasn't in control, and this fact, together with the trauma which had been dealt to my body, might mean that I really wouldn't come back. However, it wasn't just that.

The most fundamental reason I felt so upset leaving my wife was that this incident had shown me that I wanted to live and reminded me how very much I loved her and could not bear the thought of leaving her behind.

For all the years that I had been depressed, I don't believe that I had ever reached what some call 'rock bottom'. This trauma, I have since rationalised, was my rock bottom – or had certainly taken me the closest I have ever been to that awful place, although there have been times since then that have taken me right back there, which I will talk about in the third part of this story. However, this incident was my 'wake-up call', the smell of that proverbial coffee that is supposed to bring a person around from their torpor – and it had done just that.

SIX

TO THE OPERATING THEATRE...
AND DON'T SPARE THE COFFIN!

The ride down to the operating theatre on board the Flying A&E Bed, was, of course, memorable. It turned out to be a surreal experience.

It was memorable for two reasons. Firstly, I had never done it before. Secondly, I met another trolley head-on in the corridor directly outside the entrance doors to the operating theatre area.

You might think, so what? I hadn't been paying too much attention to the journey to the operating theatre before this near collision happened. My mind was full of my wife, and our dog, Gracie. They were all my family, not having any children. Not to mention the all-pervading dread of what lay ahead.

We pulled up sharply outside the theatre, causing me to raise my whirring head off the pillow. I immediately wished that I hadn't done so. Within touching distance to my left, sat a standard hospital issue white metal coffin on board the other trolley.

I had almost had a head-on collision with a

cadaver – if the coffin was occupied, of course. I remember thinking, *Christ, is this an omen?* Then, immediately and with perverse humour, the thought occurred to me that whoever the poor bugger was in there was in worse shape than me... at that immediate moment, anyway.

SEVEN
MEETING 'EDDIE THE ENDOSCOPE' AND THEN OBLIVION

A brief word on endoscopies before I continue. I believe that my life-long dread of having this procedure was justified. I found having one is really very unpleasant, so if you can avoid having one as much as possible by living a life clean of booze, I would advise you to do so. I wasn't aware of the endoscopies that I had at this time because I was anaesthetised, but for a subsequent check-up, some months later, I was fully awake.

On this later occasion, I was extremely nervous, not only because I would be awake, but I was experiencing additional anxiety, as it had been during one of the endoscopies I had in Treliske Hospital, the previous November, that the biggest of my life-threatening bleeds was triggered.

For this check-up, knowing that being anaesthetised wasn't going to be an option, I asked the nurse for the maximum of everything she could give me by way of making this procedure less dreadful. "You can have anything you like Luv." she lied.

"Great. Can you put me out then?" I ventured to ask one more time, knowing what the answer would be. "Can't do that Luv." At least she smiled benevolently when she confirmed what I already knew. The consent form which I signed as 'the Patient' stated that I could receive a throat numbing spray or a mild sedative. There was a separate box on the consent form for masochists to tick and sign who wanted neither of these options. Apparently such people do exist. I asked the nurse why it was only one or the other and not both of these pacifiers that were available to the patient. "You can have anything you like Luv." she repeated, almost robotically. In that case, I ordered the throat numbing spray and the sedative from the menu. Some people who had contributed to an online forum I had looked at previously, claimed that when they had the sedative they were 'floating' so much they had hardly been aware of anything going on during the procedure, and that it had been all over almost without them knowing it had even begun. Yeah...

Even with the joint effects of these two pacifiers, the 'Job's Comforter' of a nurse, who stayed with me during the check-up, explained that I would still gag throughout the procedure (it is a requirement that staff be transparent with the patient, even when they are bricking it). To be fair, she wasn't exaggerating. As 'Eddie the Endoscope', as I playfully

48

dubbed the offending hosepipe-like apparatus, was shoved unceremoniously down my throat (there was no mucking about exchanging social niceties with the doctor), was guided into my guts, and when he was being withdrawn from them, I gagged like fury. The Linda Lovelace guide to deep-throat fellatio I had read in preparation for the ordeal hadn't helped.

I gagged and gagged and gagged, uncontrollably, silently praying that this wouldn't start my bleeding again. It didn't, and the doctor conducting the procedure confirmed that the remaining varices were shrinking, and all looked to be healing fine, although I did have a hiatus hernia apparently. It was over! I leapt from the trolley on which I had been lying for the procedure (the sedative I had received hadn't even touched the sides) and I found my wife in the waiting room to go home. "How did it go?" she asked.

"It was nothing really," I replied, lying nonchalantly. Actually, I don't think that I was given the sedative early enough for it to take effect fully before the procedure started, hence it had no real efficacy until I was on my way home, thankfully, as a passenger, in the car!

By the way, when you are told that the endoscope is 'no thicker than the width of my little finger', as the nurse shows you her dainty little pinkie, don't believe it. If she'd had the little fingers of King Kong, that might have been a fairer comparative description.

* * *

Back to November 2015. The anaesthetist's name was Robert. He asked for me to be positioned on the operating table on my back, with my head supported at the neck, tilted as far back as possible over the end of the table where he was sat. This would allow access for Eddie the Endoscope, I supposed. Robert was sat immediately behind my tilted-back head.

I can only assume that I was placed in this position for safety and technical reasons since I wouldn't be conscious during the procedure. For the later check-up endoscopy in September 2016, I was lying on my side with my head level looking at the doctor shoving this anaconda down me and watching my innards being revealed on the video monitor in front of my face. I don't think that I should have been able to see my insides but to me, as a layman, they looked OK.

Anyway, looking upside down at Robert's crotch, while he delivered me the knockout anaesthetic punch: that's the last thing I remember until I was brought around eight days later. Most of the following chapter is an excerpt of what my wife diarised during my stay in hospital, including what she recalls was explained to her by the clinical team over the course of the next eight days. I have, therefore, used her words extensively in the following chapter.

EIGHT

"YOUR HUSBAND IS QUITE A UNIT"

Before giving way to my wife's contemporary notes, I should explain briefly, and as best as I can, what the TIPSS procedure is, as I have alluded to it previously and will be mentioning it again throughout this chapter.

This explanation has been written by a layperson and, as such, may not be 100% accurate. TIPSS stands for Transjugular Intrahepatic Porto Systemic Shunt. My drinking had caused my liver to become cirrhotic. As a consequence of the condition of my liver, I was also affected by what is known as 'portal hypertension'. As most of us are aware, hypertension is raised blood pressure. In this case, the pressure of the blood inside the portal vein, which is the main blood vessel in the liver, is raised. The pressure in my portal vein had increased because my blood was finding it more and more difficult to pass through the increased resistance of toughened cirrhotic scarred liver tissue.

Consequently, blood finds the path of least

resistance and new blood vessels, known as varices, develop to bypass the liver. Commonly, these varices extend into the oesophagus. They become twisted, knotted and fragile, just like varicose veins in the legs. Being fragile, these veins are prone to bleeding. The extent of the bleeding from varices can be minor, causing anaemia, or major, causing a haemorrhage. Blood is passed through the person's bowels or it is vomited. The blood passed in stools usually causes them to take on a very dark green-black colour.

Looking back, I had been passing blood in my stools for some considerable time, although I was ignorant of the meaning of the dark green-black warning signs. Until I started vomiting copious volumes of blood, I was unaware that I had a cirrhotic liver. Of course, I knew that I was an alcoholic, but apart from the colour of my poo, which I didn't understand, I had no other symptoms of cirrhosis such as ascites (a build-up of fluid in the abdomen), and encephalopathy (the disturbance of brain function caused by toxins remaining in the blood due to poor liver function). The discussions I had previously had with GPs due to the poor liver function, had never raised the possibility of cirrhosis, merely that my liver was having to work too hard.

However, once I had started to vomit blood, the bleeding of my varices had become a medical emergency. During the endoscopies I had, the clinical team at Treliske were able to identify the cause, site and extent of the bleeding but were unable to stop it, though it must be understood, this was not for the want of them trying and re-trying. Due to the severity of my bleeding, the use of intravenous drugs, such as Glypressin or Octreotide, were ruled out immediately. The team tried the standard approach of banding the varices in conjunction with a balloon tamponade several times but to no avail. Therefore, as I mentioned earlier, there were two options remaining for me – the TIPSS procedure or a liver transplant. As a transplant in time to save my life was highly unlikely, the only hope of saving me was to have a shunt inserted into my liver through the TIPSS procedure. However, for this procedure to be carried out I would need to be transferred to Derriford Hospital in Devon, in the company of a scrubbed surgeon and nurse in case I took a turn for the worse.

Shunting involves the joining of two veins. During the TIPSS procedure a tract is created within the liver to connect the portal vein (the vein that carries blood from the digestive organs to the liver) to one of the hepatic veins (one of the three veins that carry blood away from the liver back to the heart). This connection is kept open by the placement of a small, tubular metal device known as a shunt. This procedure lowers the portal hypertension to a level where the bleeding can be stopped.

The TIPSS procedure is not without its complications, however. One of these is hepatic encephalopathy whereby the person becomes confused. This is because the liver cannot filter toxins from the blood as it normally would. Following the TIPSS procedure, blood, and the toxins being carried by it, bypass the liver and are free to course through the body where they can play havoc with the electrical activity of the brain. Indeed, a great deal of Part Two of this story is concerned with the effects of my temporary hepatic encephalopathy.

I should also explain why I entitled this chapter, 'Your Husband is Quite a Unit'. This was a description of me, which was said to my wife by one of the doctors who was looking after me in my induced coma.

Apparently, my face, hands and feet had become swollen to the point that I would have made even the Michelin Man look like a 'size o'. In a perverse sense, I wish that my wife had taken a photograph of me when I was like this, as apparently, I was unrecognisable. It is quite common though for patients in Intensive Care Unit (ICU) to swell up in this way, caused by a build-up of fluids in the body.

Kev sedated completely for endoscopy.

Advised quite some time later by liver consultant that damage appears to have been caused primarily by alcohol abuse and that during the procedure, Kev had further major bleed, so had been put on ventilator to assist him with his breathing. Further blood given. Advised that 'bands' would be used to support the vein that was bleeding, plus balloon to be inflated to stem the flow of blood. Transferred to Intensive Care Unit.

After ensuring that Kev was as safe as could be, I was accompanied to car park to find car, as I was not aware of any charges when I arrived, so was expecting car to have been clamped possibly. Thankfully, it was fine – I was lucky. Made my way, as I thought back to Porthleven – went back and forth for fifteen minutes or so, then got my bearings and travelled back to the cottage, passing various firework displays on way back. Worried about Kev – worried about Gracie being left for so long, with fireworks being sent off (nine hours). She was fine. Took her out for quick walk, and then fed her. Made myself sandwich, but unable to eat it – going down in lumps. Gracie slept with me on bed for company. Rang later – he was comfortable.

Rang hospital – when tube taken from nose with balloon attached, further bleeding occurred, so would reinsert for a further twenty-four hours. Still on ventilator.

Rang holiday cottage company – explained situation re: Kev, and Gracie being left alone at property (as this did not comply with the terms of the rental) – asked if I could call for clean bedding/towels etc. as we were going into the second week of our rental and my cousin Adrian and his partner Helen were due to visit. Fine with that – asked if there was anything they could do.

Visited the hospital. Kev sent for CT scan to check on extent of damage to liver. Spoke to consultant and anaesthetist – liver is not as damaged as they had first suspected, but he would need to stop drinking completely if he was to make a complete recovery.

Gracie OK when I got back – had left her for six hours today. Took her for quick walk, and then fed her. Rang Adrian at pub to advise I was home.

Adrian and Helen arrived teatime. I was so pleased to see them, as it had been frightening and lonely being on my own, although at least overnight, I had Gracie with me. Adrian and I took Gracie out for a walk – while he called into Chinese and the chip shop for food for us all. Gracie settled well with Ade and Helen.

Gracie slept on the bed with me.

Rang hospital – will check later and if all OK, will take out ventilator.

Rang holiday cottage company for spare key for Ade and Helen – I called over to fetch it.

Left Gracie with Ade and Helen – they were going to St. Ives. She was fine – had asked to be picked up onto lap when they sat outside The Sloop pub. It was decided that when they leave to go home, they take Gracie with them, as it would be one thing less for me to worry about.

Visited – spoke to consultant – took Kev for further endoscopy to check on bleed. All looking better than it was yesterday. Part of the bleed yesterday had been caused by the bands they had put on the vein, plus the balloon had slipped. Intending to take him off drugs keeping him asleep, can then remove ventilator. If all OK, will be moved to specialist gastro-hepatology ward.

Ventilator removed. Within ten to fifteen minutes, Kev asking for water – drank several cups one after another. Unable to speak, as throat sore from ventilator – getting frustrated as I could not understand what he was trying to say to me. Did say, "I want to go home.", and "I want my dog."

Left hospital feeling so much better and positive for Kev.

Rang hospital – expecting positive continuation of yesterday, but instead, he had not had a good night, and two further bleeds this morning, so further endoscopy to be done. Ventilator reinserted.

Left Gracie with Ade and Helen – after spending the day in Cornwall, they were going to drop Gracie off at Jayne's on way home.

Visited hospital. Despite doctors being positive, Kev continued bleeding. Was advised that if bleed could not be stopped, they could not continue to give him further blood transfusions, as had eight-plus already. He will need to be transferred to Derriford Hospital in Plymouth for 'TIPSS' procedure, as that would be only other option if bleeding continued. Told about The Lodge (B&B) by the consultant.

Consultant advised me about the procedure, and that due to most of the toxins floating around the body, instead of processed by the liver, Kev may remain confused for a while, due to ammonia, etc. not being processed by the liver.

Advised by nurse to stay at hospital overnight as Kev really poorly. Stayed by his bedside until late, then nurse managed to find me toothpaste / brush / deodorant / towel as I had not brought anything with me. Slept on settee in visitors' waiting room, but every time I heard footsteps, kept thinking someone was coming to fetch me. My phone battery was waning, but nurse with Kev managed to borrow a charger from one of the doctors for me.

Contacted the holiday cottage company owner to advise that Kev was going to be transferred to Derriford Hospital tomorrow and that I would no longer require the cottage from then on.

9/11/15

Got up at 6am. Checked that Kev OK and that the plan was still for him to be transferred to Plymouth.

Visited Kev. Left hospital and returned to cottage to pack up belongings / food etc. Packed up car. Left cottage and returned to hospital.

Took staff a few hours to get equipment, etc. ready for Kev to be safely transported to Plymouth, as he must be completely stable before he could go. Late morning / lunchtime – Kev taken by ambulance to Plymouth – blue lighted all the way – scrubbed doctor and nurse on board. Ambulance driver advised he would ring me when they had arrived safely at Plymouth ICU.

Booked in to The Lodge for a few days, as suggested by consultant. When I got there, unpacked quickly, plus took all the food stuffs brought from the holiday cottage and put them in the fridge-freezer at the B&B, and then walked to Derriford Hospital. [The Lodge is a Bed and Breakfast establishment with a difference. It caters primarily for relatives (and patients) visiting Derriford Hospital.]

On arrival at Derriford Hospital, Kev was placed in his own room within the Intensive Care Unit. So many tubes, leads, and equipment hooked up to him. Stayed for a few hours then left. My sister Kath arriving from Cardiff to spend a few days with me.

Rang Kev's room. Had reasonably comfortable night – due to have TIPSS procedure this morning. Visited hospital. TIPSS procedure carried out – all OK. Kev stable, but slight problem with right lung – may have ingested some blood. May need fibre optic camera inserted into lung tomorrow to check extent of it. Due to have feeding tube inserted – hoping this will not cause further bleed.

Tried to take Kev off ventilator, but blood pressure too high, so had to keep him anaesthetised. Will check everything again tomorrow, but if OK, may be able to transfer him to Royal Glamorgan Hospital, Llantrisant, by specialist ambulance. No beds available there today, but if all OK, will try again tomorrow.

Rang hospital. Kev had stable night. Nurse just changing lines, which will take a few hours, there are so many. Will visit later. Going to try to bring Kev around later.

Visited – Kev's lung has been cleared. Just reducing sedation gradually – no further news so unlikely to be transferred to Royal Glamorgan Hospital today.

Taken off sedation, waiting until fully conscious. Hopefully will then remove ventilator and will either arrange transfer to a ward here or to Royal Glamorgan on 13/11.

Visited morning – ventilator to be removed.

Despite ventilator being removed, nurse could not get much reaction from him. He was asked to poke out his tongue, wiggle his toes, grip her hand with his. I continually tried for some time to get him to do any of these. Doctor arrived – he gripped Kev by the neck – Kev winced, and then did as he was asked with tongue, toes and hands. As soon as it appeared Kev was stable, Kath left to go home.

On advice, extended my stay at The Lodge for a further week.

At later visit pm. – Kev not responsive – so doctor asked for Kev to have scan of brain activity (via thirty-plus electrodes attached by glue to head), to check to see if he has had any seizures. If he has, the doctor advised that they can sort that out. It could also be a build-up of ammonia, as the liver is not now filtering all waste products due to stent implanted during TIPSS procedure. This may take some time to clear and they are going to check if this is the case. He may therefore need to go back on the ventilator. The doctor advised he will stay in the Intensive Care Unit for a few more days if he improves – if not and longer-term treatment is needed, they will get him transferred closer to home. Will know more tomorrow.

13/11/15

Kev more responsive today, although not yet fully awake – very drowsy. Off main oxygen supply, now on lesser-pressured oxygen. Kev managed to pull out feeding tube earlier, so had to have another x-ray, but all was OK. EEG is fine, so no seizures. May be transferred to a ward tomorrow but will need to see how things are tomorrow.

NINE

THE 8-DAY LONELY PLANET GUIDE TO
COMA AND INTENSIVE CARE

Eight days of nothingness.

PART TWO

MOVING TO MARLBOROUGH WARD

TEN

I WAS LOST SOMEWHERE…

Before I go any further with my story, I feel I should say something about the writing of Part Two. I wanted Part Two of the story to provide something of a comedic and hopeful counterpoint to the darkness and fear of Part One.

As it turned out, Part Two was extremely difficult to write. This took me by surprise, as I thought that Part One would be more difficult due to reliving the pain of almost losing my life.

Because of writing this story, I now believe that writing something 'funny' is an inherently difficult skill to master, and trying to mix seriousness with funniness is even more difficult. I found great difficulty in striking the right balance between the counterpoints of dark and light. However, I had to achieve this in order to give the reader (and me) a break from all the heavy stuff I was bringing to the surface and redepositing on the page; while conveying the comedy which is inherent in the human condition, sometimes even at its lowest points.

In creating a lighter counterpoint to the first part of the story, I also had to ensure that the underlying seriousness and sadness of the situation was not lost as the cause of the comedy. Therefore, it was difficult to incorporate just the right amount of pathos into the retelling of the events contained in Part Two. I hope that in the end I did this justice. I guess you will have to decide that.

The other dimension I had to keep in mind was that, in these days of political correctness, a writer of anything vaguely comedic is expected to be careful not to upset or offend others' sensitivities. I must confess that political correctness is something for which I have little or no time. Indeed, I view it as nothing more than an irritating hindrance to effective communication. However, this is not the place to debate the inanity of political correctness, and whether it has gone mad or otherwise. Suffice to say here that I have written an honest account of what happened to me while I was recovering on Marlborough Ward at Derriford Hospital.

* * *

The life-saving TIPSS procedure I underwent at Derriford Hospital was physically successful, in that it staunched the bleeding and removed from me the immediate danger of my demise.

My mind, however, had gone elsewhere due to the complication of hepatic encephalopathy, and it was a worrying time for my poor wife, waiting for it to come back... if it ever would, and hoping that it would bring me back with it. I had gone to sleep in Cornwall and woken up in Devon, but it could have been Timbuktu for all I knew. I didn't know what the hell was going on. I had woken up and found myself trapped.

I say trapped because physically I was. I was disconnected from the outside world while being securely connected to all sorts of equipment, feeds and drips in this alien place I had woken up. They were giving me countless drugs all day long it seemed. I was constantly at the mercy of staff wanting to take samples from me, and readings of my blood pressure and oxygen saturation levels. Thankfully, my sense of humour was never far from me. Once, when asked for yet another blood sample, I said "Carry on. Take as much as you like, I don't know whose it is!"

I was wearing only surgical stockings, incontinence pants and a hospital issue gown. I was incontinent, which meant I could not go anywhere, even as far as the toilet off the ward thoroughfare immediately to the right of my bed. I had no strength to stand up, let alone walk. I didn't know who I was, where I was, or what I was doing. I didn't have a watch to tell what time of day it was. I couldn't move or go anywhere for all this. I would come to realise, almost anew every day, this 'imprisonment', over and over again during the coming weeks. I was constantly wanting to leave, and attempting to get out of bed to do so, only to be pushed (very gently) back onto my bed by the ever observant, present and yet wonderful 'prison guards'. I was in a nightmarish world in which I had no control over my body or mind. I felt lost, alone, vulnerable, and frightened, somewhere which was devoid of all that was familiar to me.

Although still heavily drugged, receiving medication to detoxify me, gently wean me off the booze (or help me to forget about her) and treat the delirium tremens, I vaguely recall a conversation between my wife and a doctor taking place in which it was agreed that I would be discharged from Intensive Care and transferred to a bed on Derriford Hospital's Marlborough Ward.

The staff on the ward specialised in treating people like me. People who had ended up acutely ill, and/or their health in crisis because of alcohol, or some other 'substance misuse' – to use the politically correct euphemism. I encountered, as I came to realise later, people being cared for on the ward who were in far worse states than I was in by now. The immediate danger to my life had passed. Although I was still far from well, I could start to bleed again at any point, and therefore not out of the dark woods yet. More about that to come.

No. On the ward there were poor people in the beds next to mine, and all around me, who had no chance of making anything like a full recovery, physically or mentally. Their bodies and brains had been wrecked by their addictions and habits. I now realise that the majority of my fellow in-patients on

Marlborough Ward were suffering the long-term physical and mental health conditions caused by years and years of alcoholism.

Our community on Marlborough Ward consisted of a mixed bunch, again emphasising the fact that alcoholism is a humanity-levelling affliction.

There were undoubtedly some hitherto high functioning alcoholics, like me, professional people who had been holding down responsible well-paid careers, who's last drink had proved the one too many for their bodies to function with anymore; others were completely gaga (temporarily and permanently), some were homeless drinkers, off the street, now facing yet another crisis in their lives. Where would they go when they were 'fit' enough to be discharged from hospital? I was extremely lucky, once strong enough to leave hospital, I would return to my comfortable, warm, dry home, and eventually, if I wanted to, my comfortable well-paid job.

Some of us had alcoholic dementia, I think it's called Korsakoff-Wernicke Disease. Others, like me, were suffering the effects of temporary hepatic encephalopathy, where all the toxins that a cirrhotic liver cannot process, course through the blood system and wreak havoc with the brain and, therefore, mental capacity.

I had the latter of these brain conditions in a transient sense, caused by the stent implanted in my liver through the TIPSS procedure, by-passing the blood supply of my liver and my blood therefore not being filtered as effectively as it once used to be. I suffered with this for about two weeks. Hence my confused state while on Marlborough Ward. My clinical team prescribed medication for it immediately in the form of, of all things, a strong laxative, called Lactulose and high dosages of Thiamine / Vitamin B1. I will continue to take it, albeit now at lower dosages, for the rest of my life, lest the condition returns. It was, nonetheless a terrifying two-week vacation to horrorland where the excursions were not optional, and I was not accompanied by an appealing tour guide. However, in retrospect, these two weeks or so, without mental capacity, or at best with only fluctuating capacity, provided me with a fascinating, if somewhat disturbing, partial insight into perhaps what it is like when dementia starts to loosen one's grip on reality.

Some of my ward-fellows were alternately abusive to the staff who were caring for them, and then pathetically needy in their ways. One poor chap wanted, no needed and insisted, that the nurses tuck him in to his bed at night, or any other time of the day he wanted to go to sleep. His requests for tucking in were, therefore, pretty constant as he, like the rest of us, spent most of his day in bed. They were usually preceded by an outburst of foul language and name calling directed at the nurse and care staff and then this pathetic neediness.

I tried several times to abscond from 'Alcitraz'. I always failed in my attempts, of course. During my best attempt, I fell from the bedrail, having climbed atop of it, onto the ward floor, which I will expand upon later. I had cot sides fitted to both sides of my bed because the nurses and carers became wise to the antics I would adopt as a prelude to trying to get out of bed when I shouldn't be. For example, I would always take the bedclothes off the left side of my body, professing to be too warm, while edging off the bed and ending up in a heap. There I was thinking I was being subtle!

However, one of us did successfully abscond. He was 'the one that got away', to slip into prisoner of war analogies. He not only made it out of Marlborough Ward, but clear of the hospital entirely. He was picked up by the police, his papers not being in order, a couple of days later somewhere in Plymouth heading for Switzerland and returned to the 'Stalag'. He kept on trying to escape again and again though. I thought of him as our very own Squadron Leader Bartlett, or Big X, as he was known in *The Great Escape*. However, he was often upset and in tears because he didn't understand why he was in hospital, and why he was not allowed to leave when he wanted to. Bizarrely, I understood why he couldn't leave, but I didn't understand why I couldn't leave. However, my confusion was only temporary, while his was permanent alcoholic dementia. This chap was, for the most part, a quietly and very well-spoken gent. Looking back, I think that he had been rather 'well-to-do' at some point earlier in his life. Possibly the booze had taken his social standing away from him, like it had his identity by this stage. It was sad to see and hear him reduced to splenetic outbursts of truly foul language and aggressiveness aimed at the staff who he saw as his gaolers, not his carers, because 90% of the time he was such a gentleman and gentle man.

The guy in the bed next to me on my left was terribly and acutely ill, hence the regular curtain drawn around his cubicle preventing me from seeing the natural daylight when I first woke up on the ward. He was younger than me and a successful, professional person, an accountant I think. He did nothing but throw up blood. He had well and truly given up. He would be asked if he wanted or needed assistance to go to the toilet, give no response, then defecate in his bed as soon as the staff had left. Worst of all though, he kept throwing up the blood all over the floor around his bed. He was in receipt of much attention from the medical staff. I didn't think that he had much time left.

That's just a potted account of some of them on the ward with me. There were others who came in and out. Some of what I saw and heard should have scared, or at least disturbed me, but none of it did. I later rationalised that this was not just because I was out of my own mind most of the time, but because I was one of them. We were brothers in booze.

However, when I first found myself on Marlborough Ward, none of this occurred to me, as I didn't know where, or for that matter really, who I was.

* * *

Sometime after the conversation between my wife and the doctor about discharging me from the Intensive Care Unit, the transfer to Marlborough Ward took place. I don't know how long after the discussion it was. I don't recall the move or how I got there. I have no memory of it at all. The first thing I do remember was floating into half consciousness in a bed somewhere I didn't know. Having said that, of course, I couldn't tell you, even now, a great deal about the Intensive Care Unit I had been transferred from either, having been unconscious and, at best, semi-conscious for most of my time there.

I remember when I woke up on Marlborough Ward that I was in a busier, noisier place than before. There were lots of people around, and it was bright with artificial light. I could only see directly in front and to the right of me, where there was no natural light. The windows, I later discovered, were to the left of me at the end of the ward. Everything to the left of me was obscured by a cubicle curtain. I had been placed, I was later told, in the bed nearest to the nurses' station, where they could keep a close eye on me.

Despite there being lots of people in beds, sitting around beds and busily milling about, I didn't know or recognise anyone. I remember a feeling of incredible loneliness coming upon me. I didn't really know why I felt that way, because I didn't know where or who I was, and therefore what, where or who I was missing. It was as if I had just started my life there, in that moment of awakening in a strange bed in a strange place. I had no past.

I soon realised that the people in the beds opposite me were eating and/or being helped to eat. People in uniforms were busy about the beds, helping the sick to eat or just sitting talking to them while they fed themselves. But I had no food, and no one was acknowledging my presence, let alone talking and sitting with me. What was going on?

Of course, I didn't know that I was suffering the effects of hepatic encephalopathy. To say that I was 'confused' was an understatement. My brain was being poisoned by my own waste products, particularly ammonia. However, I remained confused, to varying degrees for pretty much for the rest of the time I was in hospital, only really starting to regain full mental capacity a couple days before being discharged, when suddenly something clicked and everything became a hell of a lot clearer.

While on Marlborough Ward, the combination of brain poisoning, medication, paranoia, delirium tremens, my fertile imagination and sleep deprivation caused me to have different imaginary (but very real to me) 'scrapes' or fictional episodes on a daily, or even more frequent basis, as I could not comprehend the passage of time. I have not recounted anywhere near all of them here as there would be too many and they would affect the balance of the overall story. 'Scrapes' is the best word to describe these fictional episodes as they were always of a dangerous, distressing or disturbing nature. However, I have to say that with hindsight the outward manifestations of what was going on in my confused mind must have been humorous to those around me who were listening or watching.

Looking back on that time, it is fascinating to me how my mind, even in the state that it was in, could still attempt to rationalise things, and lay down memories in the brain that I can still recall, seemingly in full detail, even now. I don't know how this is possible, only that I can still relate everything that was going on in my mixed-up head. I know of other people who have suffered similar effects due to urinary tract infections, for example, who have crystal-clear memories of such adventures despite having confused minds. Indeed, the incongruency of the words used in that sentence sum up the incongruency of the condition of hepatic encephalopathy as it affected me – clear memories emerging from a confused mind – inexplicable, to me anyway.

However, due to my hepatic encephalopathy, the recounting of these adventures does not bear any relation to an accurate or real timeline, as I can only be reasonably sure of the last few days on Marlborough Ward. Despite not being in anything like the full possession of my capacity, I have memories of things that either wholly happened, partially happened, or did not happen at all. However, these things were going on in my head, no doubt triggered by something innocuous happening on the ward, which morphed in my addled brain to assume greater significance. I believed at the time that all the things that will unfold from here on happened, and in some cases still did when I left hospital and continue to question the possibility of their reality even now.

ELEVEN

ANGELS AND BED-BATHS...
THAT'S BRENDA!

I don't remember how long after moving onto Marlborough Ward it had been, but it couldn't have been that long, before I encountered two lovely young ladies, both of whom were very pretty, one of them a carer, the other a nurse, who came to give me the first of many bed baths.

I had never had one before, as I had never needed one. Believe me though, between the sweatiness of being stuck in bed all day and night (at least at first) in the warm environment of a hospital ward, and the consequences of being fed a diet of liquid chemicals through a nasal tube while taking a powerful laxative, bed baths were most surely needed!

I was being cleaned up constantly following incontinence accidents. I really couldn't help it. Things would happen so quickly there wasn't even time to request a bedpan. Added to this, of course, I was incredibly confused which meant my capacity to remember when to go to the toilet, and/or summon assistance to do so, often eluded me. Sometimes, as I wasn't eating solid food, I couldn't even feel my bowels opening until the warmth of the liquid excretion had made itself apparent upon my skin and in the bed around me – not to mention the terrible smell which emanated from it, caused, no doubt, by the chemicals and medications that were being pumped into me to keep me alive at this point.

In fact, we (that is me, and the incredibly patient and lovely staff looking after me) must have set some sort of 'pit' record in the Formula One of bed changing. I could soil myself, be cleaned up and 're-Pampered', have the bed completely changed and remade (all while I was still lying on it) and soil it all over again before I even had the bed covers pulled back up. The only thing that was missing was Murray Walker's animated commentary, "...and Barnett has entered the slip lane, heading for the pits with a veritable oil slick of shit coming from his big end!"

Despite all of this, during my bed bath debut, my behavioural hardwiring kicked in. I reacted shyly, which was appropriate for me. To this day, I never like to be seen by strangers in anything less than my full regalia. I hate wearing shorts in public, for example, believing my legs to be of the same genus as 'hairius pipecleanerus'. Given my nature, therefore, I was incredibly uncomfortable, not to mention nervous, about having any part of my body, let alone my intimate bits and bobs, handled and washed by two unknown, young and, it must be said, attractive females.

Like lots of people when I'm nervous or shy, I tend to crack jokes to compensate or cover it up. However, the extreme circumstances I was in must have caused my behavioural hardwiring to go into some sort of overdrive. Here was I, this overweight fifty-year-old with a dodgy liver, the booze long ago having taken away my six-packed, ripped, racing snake physique, covered in my own faeces, teasing these poor girls like the character Fat Bastard from the Austin Powers' movies.

When they approached my bed and asked me if I would like them to give me an all-over wash, I shouted, "I'm sexy!" loudly, at the top of my croaky voice, for all to hear.

I'd even adopted the Fat Bastard Scottish accent. This was especially dangerous in my circumstances, given that the Charge Nurse on the Ward was a humungous syringe-wielding Scotsman who was responsible for giving me a particularly nasty injection into my abdomen every other day. By the way, both the syringe and the Charge Nurse were humungous!

I continued to dig myself deeper into the hole I was unwittingly preparing for myself. "Bet you two only want to get your hands on me 'cos I've got the body of Daniel Craig, don't you? If he knew what I was doing with it he'd kill me." I remembered a similar line delivered by the character Shady Tree, in relation to Rock Hudson's body, from the James Bond film, *Diamonds Are Forever.* I thought I'd best explain that, before you say you've heard that one before! The poor girls laughed with me, and continued to clean me up very gently, while taking care of what was left of my dignity, shot to bits as it was after I had done my best to assassinate it.

On a more serious note, making exaggerated claims, such as these, is a common symptom of hepatic encephalopathy.

Both these members of staff would look after me, on and off, for the entire time that I was on the Marlborough Ward, and as such they, along with several of their colleagues, became embroiled (at least in my mind) in some of the scrapes I got into on an hourly, daily and nightly basis. Only God knows what, if anything, really happened, although I really do think there is some basis in fact regarding what unfolds in this part of the story – as there is in all myths and legends, of course.

Despite never having clapped my eyes on either of them before, one of them, the young carer, looked familiar to me. In fact, she looked the spitting image of someone who had been a colleague of mine, on and off for many years, ever since that colleague had been about the same age as this carer was now – probably about twenty.

Anyway, I told the young carer that she reminded me of my colleague in work back in Wales. In fact, I added that she was now my boss. She's called Brenda, I told her further, as if these additional details would make it all make sense to this young girl. She probably didn't think any more about it.

However, by courtesy of my transient hepatic encephalopathy, over the next day or two I became convinced that the young carer was Brenda, my boss back in Wales. The real Brenda managed a team of nine, including me.

While having a subsequent bed bath, the imaginary Brenda and her colleague turned me onto my side to wash my back and rear end, shall we say. As she and her colleague were turning me over to do so, I said to the imaginary Brenda, "If you ever tell the rest of the them in the office that you've seen my bare arse and bits and pieces, I'll fucking kill you!" I should clarify at this point that I never use offensive language in front of people I don't know, and who could be offended by it, let alone direct it at anyone, like I did here, who was caring for me. I can only attribute my behaviour to my situation. However, 'Brenda' handled my confusion well, and just played along, saying she wouldn't mention a thing.

However, I became utterly convinced of this transference of identity, and at some point, during yet another bed bath, the crunch came. A different nurse had come on shift and proceeded to assist the imaginary Brenda with my bed bath. I think that she was Russian. I'll call her Nurse Rubitinski. Once they had finished my clean-up, I could see that Nurse Rubitinski was looking intently at my penis. This made me feel uncomfortable in the extreme. She stated, "Kevin, your vinky is lookink werry zaw," (I had been catheterised for quite some time by now) and then asked, in her devastatingly sexy Russian accent, "Vood you likez me to rub zum crème into eet?" Without further ado, Nurse Rubitinski proceeded to slather my inert manhood in Sudacrem.

I know, it sounds a bit like *Carry On Nurse* meets *'Allo! 'Allo!* except I was petrified. What if, "eet" reacted by rearing its ugly head? I looked at the imaginary Brenda, my eyes widening in terror. Oh my God! I freaked out. What if I get a hard-on? Brenda will tell everyone in the office! However, I had nothing to fear. Sadly, but true to what had become the norm by then, my "vinky" remained the cold, unresponsive, impassive, and useless lump of lard it had been over the last few years...

TWELVE

PARANOIA

While recovering on Marlborough Ward, I spent some considerable time experiencing dark moments in dark places. This, again, was no doubt a consequence of my hepatic encephalopathy and withdrawal from the booze.

I must say that in all the time I had been drinking, I never suffered from alcoholic paranoia or delusional disorder – at least I don't think I did. However, during this time of recovery some of what was going on in my head most certainly felt like I had now succumbed to these disorders.

A great deal of the paranoia which was now coming to the fore seemed to be connected to my wife. Looking back, I wonder if this was connected to the fear I had been experiencing for a long time during my extended bouts of depression and alcoholism, of the possible consequences of neglecting my wife. Indeed, I had on many an occasion actively encouraged my poor wife to find someone else who could give her the life she deserved, in a full and happy marriage or relationship, rather than the existence she was putting up with by being married to me. An existence that rarely revolved around anything more than my uselessness and constant helplessness.

For I don't know how many years leading up to the events of this story, I had not paid my wife sufficient attention. For example, there had been no intimacy between us for longer than I could remember, and to describe any displays of affection coming from me as fleeting would be far too generous. It wasn't that I no longer found my wife desirable, or that I didn't want to love her. On the contrary, I am a very lucky man to have been blessed with such a lovely and attractive woman to have as his wife. Unfortunately, the years of intimacy with my friend with benefits had taken their toll upon certain bodily functions. Not wishing to equate a display of affection as a necessary precursor to lovemaking, I was nevertheless afraid that if a display of affection were to possibly lead to a spontaneous act of lovemaking, I would not be able to continue. As time went by, of course, this fear led to the dearth of both simple, warm, tender affection, and the oneness and passion of lovemaking. My body had convinced my mind, and my mind had convinced my body not to start something I could not finish. Unfortunately, my wife had been drawn inside my perfectly realised vicious circle.

When I was particularly ill with depression and not in work for weeks and months on end, my wife would go to work all day and come home, dreading putting the key in the lock because she knew that the moment she stepped over the threshold, she would feel the weight of the gloom I had filled the house with. All I had done all day, every day, was brood and drink. I'd done nothing of any remotely constructive purpose.

I even found opportunity to indulge myself with my 'mistress' when ostensibly doing something for my wife. For example, I cooked my wife tea every evening during the working week but would spend an inordinate amount of time preparing something as simple as a jacket potato with cottage cheese for her in the kitchen on the ground floor of our townhouse. Why would preparing such a simple meal take me so long, and why would I insist so intently that my wife take time to relax in front of the television in the living room on the floor above? Because, on my own down there, I could secretly carry on with my mistress, spending quality time drinking deeply of her, taking her, which I should have been doing with my wife.

The secrecy was a terrible thing. It was exhausting never to be able to relax, just in case my wife would find one or all of my hidden stashes of booze. It is perhaps this secrecy, the constant deceit of my wife, of which I am most ashamed. Bottles of wine, spirits, canned beers and ciders, full and empty to varying degrees, were hidden all over the house, in the garage and in my car. It would be no exaggeration to estimate that on times there were hundreds of them. Receipts, indicating purchases of alcohol, totalling God knows how much money, were forced down the backs of furniture – hundreds of them too. I occasionally took an early morning visit to the supermarket in order to dump my empties in the recycling skips. My God, you should have seen it. I recall dumping hundreds of bottles at a time, saved up in the capacious back of my Land Rover. The crash and smash of the glass as the bottles landed in the skips made me worry about the attention I must have been drawing to myself – perhaps I did suffer from paranoia, after all. At least that was a load of evidence disposed of which my wife would never know about. Ha!

There were times I remember finding the odd wine bottle, amongst the catholic brothel menu empties, which had perhaps a third, a half, or maybe just the smallest mouthful of its contents still inside. It was like that feeling one gets upon finding a tenner in the pocket of an old coat. I would get back in the car and neck the sometimes rancid, contents. If it was foul tasting, it certainly did not bother me. A case of waste not, taste not? As I was in the car park, following the ceremonial dumping of the empties, I would pop in to the supermarket and stock up all over again for the day. Usually, I didn't even wait to get home to open what I had just purchased. I'd open it in the car while sat in the car park for ten minutes, first checking that I wasn't in view of any CCTV camera or anyone also sat in their car. If I thought I was, I would leave the bottle wrapped in the carrier bag while I took big mouthfuls, so it could not be seen.

When my wife located my latest hiding place, we would argue. She was terribly worried for me, and scared that I was taking such a self-destructive path. I argued that my privacy had been affronted. How dare she go looking for things! Isn't anything sacred anymore? Of course, I knew, even then, that she was right. I promised her again and again to curb my drinking, but I did not possess the strength to stop myself. The thought of drinking, and drinking itself, was all-consuming.

Instead, I found new places to hide my mistress from my wife. Towards the end, it became almost like a Brian Rix farce. Enter bedroom right, my wife, exit bedroom left, my little Russian tart, to be hidden in the living room behind the stereo speaker and the curtain. I congratulated myself on my ingenuity in foiling my wife's latest attempts to spoil my fun – except I wasn't having fun, I knew I was killing myself and it was all a terrible strain.

Sometimes, especially when my wife found bottles after I had made yet another promise to cut down, or at least not be so secretive, she would be upset or go very quiet.

All of this went on and on and on, and in no time, it had been like this for years. My behaviour, and the situation it caused our relationship to be in, would have tested any marriage. Indeed, I have no doubt it would have ended many. However, my truly amazing wife stuck with me. If she hadn't you wouldn't be reading this now.

* * *

Yes, the paranoia I was experiencing during withdrawal, and the confusion of hepatic encephalopathy, really did centre on my wife. This manifested itself in imaginary scenes of fear that became increasingly dramatic and elaborate, causing me to have heartrending anxiety about being separated from my wife, either out of her own choice or due to the actions of others over which I had no influence.

For instance, initially I believed that my wife had abandoned me. This thought first occurred to me one night, not long after moving onto Marlborough Ward, when probably having been asleep during visiting, I woke up to find that she was not there and I did not remember that she had been sat with me for hours earlier. I was fretting and anxiously asked one of the nurses where my wife was, as I hadn't seen her that day. "She's gone back to The Lodge," the nurse told me. Being totally disorientated, this meant nothing to me at first. However, for some reason, when I thought about the whereabouts of The Lodge, I equated it with a hotel near to where we lived in South Wales. I accused the nurse of making it up. "Why would she go to The Lodge instead of going home?" You see, I still had an idea of where 'home' was and it was only a short distance from the hotel I thought of as The Lodge. Adding to my confusion was the fact that I didn't comprehend how far away from home I was. Indeed, there were other times when I thought I was staying in a private residential care home close to where we lived. All in all, this made the nurse's answer nonsensical to me.

Not understanding what she had told me, I said to the nurse that my wife had left me. I couldn't be placated over this and was still insisting that Jan had left me the following morning, not having slept at all due to the worry of it. I plagued the Ward Sister to telephone my wife to see where she was and to have it confirmed that she had, in fact, left me. The Ward Sister said that I was being silly, and that my wife would be visiting me later on that afternoon. Of course, Jan turned up a little while later.

Not long after that though, I spent the whole of one distressing night believing that my wife had been shot and killed, en route to visiting me while I was receiving treatment at a private heart clinic in India, run by an eminent Indian doctor and her two sons. The Indian police came to the clinic to speak to the doctor to inform her that there had been a shooting, and a British woman had been killed while on her way there to visit her husband. The gunmen were still at large. Indeed, the gunmen turned up and the clinic was under siege for some hours. I became convinced that I could hear the nerve splintering sound of gunfire outside the clinic. A family feud had apparently erupted violently, and the British woman had simply become collateral damage. Jan never visited. She was the one who had been shot. I had lost her and lay in bed calling out for her all night.

Another time, we were flying back from a holiday somewhere, for some reason (but as you do) on board a billionaire's luxuriously customised private jet. My wife and I had been talking but I remember being sleepy. I fell asleep, and when I woke up she had gone (only back to The Lodge after evening visiting time had ended) but I thought something more sinister had occurred.

When I had woken up, an enormous black man in a uniform was standing over me. By 'enormous', I don't mean that he was overweight. The enormous black man was muscularly magnificent, with a viscerally intimidating bearing. The enormity of his physical presence and yet, quiet demeanour, stoked my rapidly growing paranoia about him. I glanced around me and saw that my wife was not there. I asked him if she had perhaps gone to powder her nose (powder her nose? I have never, before or since, used such an expression) before we came in to land at Heathrow. I was tired, I explained, and had been unable to stay awake for the last hour or so of the flight. Perhaps my wife had become bored and gone to use the on-board spa or have a lie down herself? She would need to come back quickly to disembark the plane with me, I added anxiously. To me, he appeared to be a bit too cagey about these matters, merely mumbling that she had "gone home" and that we should "let the lady rest". Gone home? That wasn't possible. The last thing that I remember was that we were on a jet coming in to land at Heathrow. "Let her rest"? What the hell did he mean by that?! In reality, of course, he would have been referring to the fact that my wife had gone back to The Lodge and that visiting was over for the night.

Alarm bells were now well and truly going off in my head. I had not met the enormous black man before (he was, of course, a carer) and he was soon joined by another man (another carer) whom I had also not met before. They were just carers on a different shift. However, I believed that they were both employees of our generous, or maybe not so generous, possibly sinister benefactor, who were waiting to help with our luggage when it finally emerged on the carousel.

Why had we been on that jet anyway? I couldn't remember. Christ, I hope we hadn't got caught up in some sort of trouble, Jan could be so naïve and too trusting a lot of the time! Knowing her, she'd probably agreed to something while I was sleeping. It was just like that time when we were on holiday in India, when she'd agreed with the suggestion of the taxi driver, that it would be a good idea to go and have a look at some 'antiques' while we were on our way to Mapusa Market in Goa. This was despite my most animated protestations that we couldn't and shouldn't. A whole lifetime later, and feeling that we had been kidnapped, we were 'released' from this warehouse in the middle of the 'Indian Nowhere' after finally convincing the most tenacious of salesmen that we couldn't afford £2,000 for the illegal handmade Kashmir wool / silk rug no matter how many knots per square inch it had tied into it.

Anyway, I digress by way of illustrating my wife's potentially dangerous naivety. Bizarrely, the fact that I was lying in a hospital bed in the middle of Heathrow Arrivals waiting for luggage signalled nothing out of the ordinary to me. Of course, the two male carers were just doing their jobs, cleaning me up and changing me, following yet another bout of faecal incontinence.

With still no sign of my wife coming back to join us, the alarm bells in my head were getting louder. When the enormous black man went to fetch something, I took the chance to speak to the other man about my suspicions, on the off chance that he wasn't involved in whatever it was that was so obviously going on. I spat what I had to say out as quickly as I could, lest the enormous black man returned before I had a chance to complete my sentence, "That bastard has either killed my wife or had her kidnapped!"

The other man, not only knew my name, but when he addressed me, he shortened it to my preferred diminutive. To address a patient in their preferred manner was, of course, hospital policy. However, in the circumstances as I perceived them to be, his 'familiarity' also disturbed me.

"Kev, she just went home a few minutes ago.

She'll be back tomorrow to visit you." I wouldn't have any of it.

"Look, we've just got off your boss's plane!" I gestured at the wall of the ward behind me with my thumb. In my mind's eye the wall wasn't there. Instead, there was a vast airport concourse. "How can she have gone home?"

The enormous black man then returned. I accused him directly this time. "What have you done with my wife? You've killed her, haven't you? I know!" Understandably, after I had repeated my accusation about a dozen times, and he, together with his colleague, had light-heartedly stuck to their story, the enormous black man snapped, "Look! We're only trying to help you!" I decided to let them finish whatever it was they were doing and said no more to them on the matter of my disappeared wife.

However, the enormous black man's reaction to my persistent accusations against him did not bring the necessary clarity to the situation for my confused mind, so the matter was not over as far as I was concerned. I thought quickly about how I would try to follow in the tracks of whoever had taken my wife, either dead or alive, murdered or kidnapped, from the airport. I settled on the idea of making good my escape through customs, or wherever I had to go to find the exit, get in my Land Rover (my beloved car was, of course, faithfully waiting for me outside the terminal building) and on the trail of the bastards who were responsible – all while dressed only in my longsuffering incontinence pants, DVT (deep vein thrombosis) stockings and a hospital gown. Not to mention that I was still connected by my nose to the hospital oxygen supply, a tube from the stand with my liquid chemical food passing directly in to my stomach, and to the bed by a large bag of piss, a catheter, and my penis.

These were not obstacles to me! In fact, I'd totally forgotten that I had all these other encumbrances preventing me from escaping to freedom and effecting the rescue of my wife – if she was still alive. No. The first, and trickiest manoeuvre was simply to get out of bed. As I hadn't long left Intensive Care, and due to my ongoing confused state and propensity to attempt absconding, it had been decided that it would be safer for me to have bedrails put up around me.

Of course, in my confusion I believed that the enormous black man and his sidekick, (both of whom were now conspicuous by their absence, no doubt having left in a hurry to join up with their gang), had confined me with this 'fence thing' to stop me from setting off in pursuit of my wife and her killers or kidnappers. I was conscious of the time ticking away and the trail going cold, but I had to time my escape with military precision.

From my bed, I was timing these women in different coloured uniforms who had gathered around a desk in front of an office (this was, in fact, the nurses' station) just to the right of me in the 'terminal building'. Who were they and what were they doing? I asked myself. Must be something to do with Jan's disappearance. They seemed to be popping in and out of that office every now and then for a minute or two. If I timed it just right, I should have enough time to be able to climb over this bloody fence around me, get passed that desk while they are in the office behind it, and out of the building to my waiting Land Rover, whereupon the keys to said vehicle would spontaneously and miraculously appear in my hand.

I waited for the women to go into the office a couple more times, and on the third occasion I made my bid for freedom. While I was observing the uniformed ladies' ingress and egress of the office behind the desk, and in preparation for mounting the bedrail, I had streamlined all the various leads and tubes attaching me to equipment around my bed. That way I hoped to minimise the possibility of getting caught up in them as I went 'over the top'.

I grabbed the rail and edged over to it, putting my legs over it first, hoping to somehow lift myself onto it into a sitting position and then just slide off, side-saddle fashion. I tried a few times but couldn't manage it from that angle. My change of approach was to align myself with the rail along the full length of the bed, from which position I straddled the rail, like Slim Pickens straddling the bomb as it dropped from his B52 bomber at the conclusion of *Dr. Strangelove*. Having got face down on top of the rail, I had two options, both of which involved just letting go and hoping for the best. I could either fall back into bed with its lovely pressure-relieving mattress or fall onto the hard floor. Well, I had come this far, and I couldn't afford to waste any more time, or I'd never catch up with the bastards who had taken my wife. So, I let go and fell with a 'thwack', face down onto the floor. I was hardly cat-like stealth in action. It didn't hurt though. I was far too confused to recognise physical pain, not to mention highly focused on getting away.

However, the commotion I had caused by dropping from the bedrail had alerted the uniformed women. They were on to me and my escape attempt was thwarted. Two of them, like storm troopers, came running over to me, as I lay on the hard floor too weak to be able to get to my knees, let alone my feet. I was reminded by the nurse with the moustache and German accent, straight out of BBC central casting, (only kidding, she wasn't really, although as far as I was concerned in that moment, her manner was) that I was barely a couple of days out of Intensive Care, and that if I tried to escape again she would have me restrained or placed in solitary confinement until I curbed my behaviour. I proudly replied that I knew my rights under the Geneva Convention (actually I think I made it quite clear that I knew my rights around being restrained and liberty-deprived), and that she would find that most difficult to do, adding that we had laws in this country to protect vulnerable people from being held against their will. I was right, of course, up to a point. That point being that I wasn't in full possession of my faculties, and it probably wouldn't have taken a great deal more of my shenanigans for me to have had my liberty legally deprived, or worse, be sectioned under the Mental Health Act.

I explained that I was Kevin Barnett and very important (I didn't know that they already knew me). I still didn't know who they were, or where I was, or why I was there) and what had happened leading up to my ending up on the floor. I was afraid that my wife had been killed or kidnapped by the two men, I told them. Did you know that one of them was an enormous black man, I asked? I needed to give chase to him. I was calmed down, put back into bed, and one of the uniformed women sat and talked with me well into the night. Just before I left hospital, I found out from her that she had done this for me on several occasions when I was having a bad night. I simply can't remember the other times, I must have been so far out of it. In my opinion, that's why nurses are sometimes, quite rightly, referred to as 'angels'.

THIRTEEN
IMAGINATION AND SLEEP DEPRIVATION

I have been told over the years that I have an extremely vivid imagination. In addition to connecting my feelings of guilt and regret over how I had been spoiling my wife's life, the paranoia I was now exhibiting was probably feeding my imagination and growing stronger while I was without the capacity to rationalise what was going on around me.

Added to this I almost wasn't sleeping at all. I hadn't really had a good night's sleep in years, but since moving to Marlborough Ward my insomnia just got worse. I have wondered since if sleep deprivation also contributed to my confused state of mind during this initial period of convalescence.

I had fitfully dozed off again during visiting, and my wife had left me sleeping (as she always has and still does if she can so that I can snatch even the smallest amount of sleep whenever it comes upon me) without waking me to say goodnight. When I awoke, I was convinced that I was the central figure in an ancient shaman ritual that one of my doctors wanted to try out on a patient in his care, following a study trip relating to the medicine of certain Native North American people.

I recall being 'prepared' to receive the ministrations of the shaman doctor. In reality, of course, I was probably just receiving my usual care: my prescribed medication, having my nasal food tube flushed out and fresh supplies of purple liquid chemical goo hooked up to me. In my confused mind, I awaited the arrival of the shaman doctor who was to be brought, with hushed, subdued ceremony and reverence, to my bedside by my regular doctor. The ward was now almost in complete darkness, save for the thoroughfare lighting to the right of my bed. I imagined that all my bedbound ward-fellows were watching my bed intently, their dead eyes wide and mouths set almost rictus-like but with eager anticipation of whatever was about to happen to me.

This felt spooky. I had convinced myself that I was unable to move a single muscle of my body. I was gripped, briefly, by a paralysis of fear. It was highly atmospheric, as if the very air around me was electrically charged. I swear that I could hear the wind howling outside. Had the approaching shaman doctor summoned a wind god or spirit? In the reality of Devon, far away from the fantasy Native American Reservation, a real storm named Barney, the second of the winter of 2015, was actually raging outside the hospital as I lay prone in my bed, awaiting whatever was going to be done to me. It could well have been Storm Barney that was tripping my imagination into overdrive, providing the cinematic sound effects to my shaman fantasy.

Apart from the howling wind outside, the ritual was proceeding in hushed silence inside the hospital. In the subdued light, I could make out the shadows of figures who I recognised as people I had been seeing a lot of recently. They were behaving differently though, swooping and gliding around me like silent spectres. Occasionally, their faces, which had become ghoulishly distorted and luminescent in the semi-darkness, would materialise immediately in front of mine, their mouths open wide like my bedded ward-fellows in silent rictus. They made no sounds, and the whole scene was devoid of sounds. It was almost as if the ward had become a vacuum, in and across which no sound could exist or travel. There was just the howling wind outside and the pounding of my heart against the wall of my chest. Then the horrifying thought occurred to me that this ritual could well conclude with my sacrificial death. I was screaming out, hoarsely, "I'm frightened! They're holding me against my will." and "I'm going to be killed." I had become desperate to see my wife who was living in the apartment down the spiral staircase in the corner of the room. I pleaded with whoever would listen, to be allowed to go to her. I remember calling out into the semi-darkness of the ward to her that they wouldn't let me go, they were going to kill me, and not for her to think that I didn't want to be with her.

The fact that I had very little voice at this time added to my frustration and agitation. My voice had not yet recovered from me being ventilated for a protracted period before coming around from my induced coma. My throat was very sore and my voice, at times, practically non-existent. I was therefore putting all the necessary physical effort in my desperation here to shout, but very little sound was coming out of my mouth.

Of course, there was no ritual, but nevertheless, I was having a night filled with terrors. I was physically very uncomfortable too. In addition to the spooky shaman ritual and not being allowed to visit my wife in her apartment down the spiral staircase, I was having difficulty relieving my bladder. It was suddenly all becoming too much for me. I was starting to panic as I could feel myself filling up with boiling urine, which seemingly could not be released. I asked for help and was told to just go to the toilet through the catheter, but I had become convinced that it was not working. The nurse had no choice but to check if the catheter was functioning. I begged her to take it out of me, it was causing me so much irritation; and the pain in my bladder and kidneys from the building pressure was becoming unbearable. My eyes must have been bulging in my head. I was sweating profusely I was so hot, and felt restricted and claustrophobic, even by the tight DVT stockings I still had on. The nurse refused to remove the tight stockings, and was reluctant to remove the catheter, as she would have to reinsert a new one, even though I was in such a state. As it happens, she was the only nurse on duty that night and was from an agency. Not only was I 'kicking off' but, by now, so were some of the others on the ward. It may well have been that my behaviour was causing everyone to become unsettled – almost as if my highly energetic but disturbed brainwaves were being telekinetically transmitted to all on the ward.

The agency nurse was obviously harassed, but did remove my catheter and brought me a cardboard bottle to relieve myself in. This I did with enormous relief. Relief which was so palpable that it made my whole body shake, as my bladder emptied itself of its high pressure, steaming hot contents. She asked me if that was better, to which I replied, with watering eyes, "Oh, Yesssss!" The nurse then showed me the empty urine bottle. I had just had a 'phantom pee'. The nurse reinserted the catheter, though I asked her not to. This caused me to become 'arsey', to use the vernacular. My agitation reached new heights as I thrashed about in bed unable to cope with the suffocation of what I saw only as my entrapment.

In the end, a doctor was summoned, and I was injected with something. I assume that the hypodermic syringe contained diazepam, or the like, although I do not recall being told this. I was told though, or rather had it shouted at me, that it would quickly calm me down and I would be able to sleep in minutes. The injection had little or no effect and my agitation raged on. The nurse summoned the doctor over, as she was unable to do anything to placate the body of a person that had by now assumed all the characteristics of one possessed by an evil spirit (save the 360-degree head spin). I recall the doctor telling the nurse that the injection I had earlier should have been sufficient to settle me down and that she really shouldn't give me another one. However, I pleaded with the doctor to give me a further shot, which she did. My body and mind continued to fight against it, but eventually the second injection worked, and I became acquiescent to the encouragement of the doctor and nurse to relax and fell into a chemically induced sleep.

FOURTEEN

'HOLBY CITY'

Some of what was going on in my head was actually quite funny. Here's a little foray my mind made into BBC Drama. Where the basis in reality for this episode of confusion was I still cannot explain, as I have never watched the television drama I was channelling in my mind. My wife, and one of the care workers on Marlborough Ward who looked after me, were actually involved in this episode of hepatic encephalopathy delusion.

I say I can't explain it because, unlike some of my previous episodes of delusion, I had been wide awake and was chatting to my wife, almost normally, as it took hold of me.

As I recall it, my wife was sat in a chair to the left of my bed. I turned to my right, glanced at what was going on in the thoroughfare between my bed and the nearby nurses' station, and then turned back to my wife and said, in a completely matter-of-fact way, something like, "I wonder if they have finished for the day now." I jerked my head back, gesturing to the assembled individuals around the nurses' station. I sensed that my wife hadn't understood or heard me properly, as my voice was still so unreliable. I, therefore, proceeded to expound upon what was perfectly clear to me and, no doubt, to everyone else except my wife it seemed. A slight note of frustrated edginess had already crept into my voice as I tried to get her to understand what I was saying. "I wonder if they've finished filming now. If they have, perhaps they've finished with me too, and I can go home for the day."

"What are you on about now – filming?" My wife said, shaking her head annoyingly and somewhat obtusely, I thought. "Filming this episode! I should get a mention in the credits this time, as I've had a speaking part." My poor wife was at a loss.

"Episode of what?" she enquired, looking intently at me. I looked at her aghast, in complete disgust and disdain. How could she not know what I, the great actor and her own husband, was working on. "Oh, come on!" I was getting more than a little tired of her pretending not to know what I was talking about. "You know full well what I'm talking about. *Holby City!* If they don't require me now that shooting is over, perhaps we can go home. That's all I'm saying. Perfectly bloody simple!"

"Kev, you're in hospital." *Why was she persisting with this childish pretence of hers, that she doesn't understand?* "Yes. I know that I'm in 'hospital'." I even did the air quotation marks at this point. "This is

Holby General." I mocked my wife, clarifying, as I thought unnecessarily, that I was indeed in the eponymous fictional hospital of the BBC television medical drama.

"You think you're in Holby City?" she questioned, maddening calmly. How much longer could she keep this nonsense up? I was incredulous by now. "What? I don't just think, I KNOW. I'm in Holby bloody City!" By now, my wife was laughing. She couldn't help it, as I was so convinced about being a character in the latest episode. Her amusement, of course, was driving me around the proverbial bend.

"Look!" I said, deciding to carry on trying to prove to her that this was a TV set, as perhaps she really didn't see things as they really were. "See those people over there. They're not *real* doctors and nurses, they're actors. Can't you see all the filming equipment – the lights, cameras and medical props?" Of course, they were real doctors, nurses and carers. What I was mistaking for lights, cameras and props was real medical equipment on stands.

I carried on at my poor wife. "The thing with you is, that you are beginning to confuse reality and fantasy." My wife was now at a loss as to how she was going to convince me that I was not an actor and not on a TV set. Spying one of my regular carers, amongst the 'actors', my wife went over to him and asked if he would come over to speak to me. "What's up then Kev?" he asked me in his broad West Country accent.

"I was just wondering if they'd finished with me for the day, and didn't need me any further, that I might go home for the evening." A perfectly reasonable proposition, I thought.

"Well the doctors have finished with you for the day and so perhaps get some rest now." he encouraged, knowing that I wasn't getting sufficient sleep.

I misunderstood this as a cue that filming had indeed finished. "Oh, right. I'll go home now then. It's Thursday night and I wanted to watch *Question Time* and *This Week*, you see. They're my favourites you know – David Dimbleby and Andrew Neil," I added, as matter-of-factly as you like.

"I'll get into terrible trouble if these doctors," he pointed to the actors, "come around tomorrow and you're not here." My carer was talking gibberish, or was he in on whatever stupid practical joke my wife was playing on me by pretending not to know I was working on Holby?

"Oh, don't worry about that." I played along and reassured him that I would be back tomorrow when shooting started again. "I mean, I only live ten minutes up the road from the studios."

"Kev, where do you think you are?" That confirmed it. He was definitely involved in my wife's stupid game. With a sigh of boredom at the banality of this idiotic charade, I reluctantly confirmed that I was "on the Holby City set at the studios in Cardiff, of course. As if you didn't know."

Like my wife, my carer had also begun to find this all very amusing. He conceded that yes, Holby City was made in Cardiff. I smiled and lifted my eyes skyward, as if vindicated. "But you're in Plymouth. Thass woi we all torx loike tha, innit." This is my written effort at describing the exaggerated West Country accent he put. "Well of course you do, it's set in Bristol."

I gave up.

It was strange because I knew by then that I had been talking through my arse. Still, I had given my poor wife some amusement amid all the worry she was going through. It was as if for the briefest moment clarity had returned. However, with that clarity came the realisation that I wouldn't get a credit for appearing in the show, and I wouldn't get to see David Dimbleby or Andrew Neil on telly in the comfort of my own home that night either. Most disappointingly, though, before my confusion took hold again, I realised that I was still not going home...

FIFTEEN
ONE LAST LONG NIGHT OF 'FUN'

I got it into my head that one of the nurses who was looking after me, and the Registrar who was attached to the Gastrointestinal and Hepatology Department (I'll refer to them as Anne and Bill) were in a relationship. Occasionally, they took patients home with them at weekends, for respite from the ward, to their house where they had a private recuperation facility.

Added to this, Anne and Bill were also both actors and Anne was an award-winning playwright and author. During the weekend away, Anne and Bill were going to start rehearsing a new play, which Anne had written. One of the other patients on the ward, in fact from the bed next to mine, would be joining us at their home this weekend. In my confused mind, he happened to be a famous actor friend of theirs who had recently had a serious relapse and was drinking heavily again. He was going to have a part in the play when it reached the stage, and so would be rehearsing with them.

Physically, Anne and Bill's famous actor friend was a lot like Ray Winstone. He looked like someone you didn't mess about with. However, whereas the real Mr. Winstone has class, this guy was without any. Needless to say, I took an instant dislike to him, and my paranoia about him grew steadily throughout this episode of confusion.

Actor?! He was nothing more than a loud-mouth ham! I couldn't understand why they were friends with him, and indeed, for some reason Anne and Bill appeared beholden to him. Although, like me, this excuse-for-an-actor was being cared for because he was an alcoholic, he was being treated to glasses of Dom Perignon with spherical pearls of green chartreuse – looking like angelica caviar. How pompous! Meanwhile, Bill offered me a lousy beer. I demurred, adding that I hadn't taken a drink for about six weeks now, thank you, and I didn't intend starting again.

In between caring for me and a few others, rehearsals with the famous actor who looked like Ray Winstone were taking place. I could hear him quite clearly in his phoney excuse for the beautifully characterful cockney accent, swearing when he fluffed his lines and demanding yet another of his pretentious drinks. I decided that his uncouth manner and disrespect towards Anne in particular warranted his death, and I had worked out how I was going to kill him.

One evening, as Anne was attending to my

purple liquid-goo food bag, I asked her if Mr. Ray Winstone's bed was electrically operated like mine was. Looking puzzled by my question, she said that it was. I confessed to her that I had had it up to here, demonstrating with my hand across my forehead, with the way he was treating her and his uncouth manner generally. It was time that somebody did something about him. Moreover, it was time that I did something about him, and I was going to.

Having ascertained that his bed was electrically operated, I asked Anne if she remembered the James Bond film, *Goldfinger*, in which oo7 killed his would-be assassin by electrocuting him in the bath? For some reason, instead of just answering my perfectly reasonable and straightforward question, she asked me why I had asked it.

"Cos I'm going to kill 'im," (pointing to the obnoxious crook in the bed next to me) "like 'e (James Bond) did in Goldfinger. When it's quiet later, I'm gonna throw my jug of water over 'is bed and watch 'im fry!" Anne didn't appear to be impressed by the intentions of my chivalric spirit, or at all bothered, either, when I carried out the assassination attempt. As I shouted "For fuck's sake shut up and show some respect!" at the top of my unreliably hoarse voice, my pathetically weak left arm's effort at hurling the water as far as Ray Winstone's bed, resulted only in a small puddle on the floor between us, which Anne, of course, then had to clean up.

As the evening wore on, I grew increasingly

concerned and annoyed that Ray Winstone was still alive and lying smugly in his bed next to mine guzzling champagne and bursting the delicate jelly chartreuse pearls in his camel-like mouth. His demands were really becoming beyond a joke and seeing that I had failed in my endeavour to kill him, I was so pleased to see that the nurses had decided to bump him off themselves. They used a concoction of vast amounts of finely ground black pepper, cayenne pepper, potent red chillies and lemon juice made into a hot drink with tea. I could hear the hitherto angels forcing this liquid, which must have been like searingly hot battery acid, down Ray Winstone's throat, as they told him they knew it was unpleasant, but it was for his own good. He was choking and gagging, and I could hear him throwing it up all over the floor, but they just kept on forcing more down him until in the end his death rattle came and then the subsequent silence signalled it was all over.

Despite my intense dislike of Ray Winstone, I thought *I wouldn't want to mess with them* – the nurses. All was silent as the nurse assassins laid him out in the bed next to me. They left the body of Mr. Winstone there in the bed, covered by a sheet. Only his blue dead feet were visible at the end of his bed. When they had finished, and turned to walk away from the bed, I winked at them to acknowledge a job well done, not only because I was pleased that they had succeeded, but also because I thought it would be in my long-term interests to stay on their good side.

Oddly enough (but then pretty much everything was odd for me at the time) the thought of having the dead body of Ray Winstone in the next bed did not bother me in the slightest. However, it seemed like some hours later, I was lying on my left side looking in the direction of the late Mr. Winstone's bed, with his corpse still lying in it, when I felt a terrific pain in my backside. Thinking back to it, and attempting to rationalise things, I think I had been given a suppository for some reason – it was almost as if a member of the nursing staff had administered it covertly while I wasn't looking, as I don't recall being told I was going to have one.

Possibly it was because my confused state was showing no signs of improvement and the daily doses of Lactulose were not clearing the toxins from my blood as efficiently as they might. Anyway, only a short time afterwards I was desperate to go to the toilet due to the burning and cramps in my abdomen. I couldn't wait for help to arrive, and soiled myself. Time for the 'bed-pit crew' to do their thing. However, while they were cleaning me up, the corpse of the counterfeit Ray Winstone suddenly started to move and groan.

If I hadn't already done so, I probably would have shit myself at the sight of the deceased Mr. Winstone raising up, Lazarus-like, to sit bolt upright in his bed. 'Ray Winstone' was actually the poor chap to the left of me on the ward I mentioned at the start of Part Two of the story. He was the accountant who was very poorly. What I had witnessed was him having one of his terrible episodes. He was having them regularly. He wasn't vomiting some spicy concoction made by the nurses to kill him, but pints of blood, like I had been a couple of weeks earlier.

Not long after having seen Ray Winstone come back to life, I fell asleep.

When I awoke, I believed that I was staying in a luxury hotel. Ray Winstone was propped upright in his bed to the left of mine. For some strange reason, I felt that I owed him an apology for trying to fry him by electrocution earlier. I started jabbering on about actors and acting, trying to find some common ground over which we might have a chat. Then I asked him if he had a spare cigarette, as I noticed he had lit up one and was puffing away merrily on it. He didn't have one for me he said and just wanted to get comfortable before the 'show' started. I didn't know anything about a show.

My carer came over to my bed to see how I was. I gestured to my left with my head and said that 'Ray' had mentioned there was to be a show tonight. I didn't know the hotel provided entertainment, I explained. My carer smirked saying that occasionally the hotel was cleared of guests for an evening, having been hired by a production company to make porn films. I could participate if I surrendered my credit card but would only be allowed to watch from the sidelines if I didn't pay up. I didn't know if I had a credit card I said, so I would just watch if I felt like it.

My carer left more than a bit pissed off that he hadn't got a payment out of me.

Now I was getting somewhere. It had taken months of undercover work to infiltrate this ring of filth, but I had finally done it. I was now Jim Bergerac, the 1980s fictional television detective from Jersey. I thought I should telephone HQ. I picked up the telephone from the side of my bed and telephoned to tell my colleagues that "the balloon had gone up" and "tonight was going to be the night" and no doubt many other similar clichés. There was no telephone, of course, merely my call bell for summoning assistance from the nurses' station. There was lots of activity going on in the room around me. They were setting up lighting and cameras, so I tried to be as discrete as possible on the telephone, lest I draw attention to myself.

My carer returned to my bedside. He looked concerned. "Have you been trying to get an outside line on your call bell again Kev, or is there something wrong?" I had in a previous episode of extreme confusion been trying to telephone the woman who was looking after our dog by using the call bell handset. On this occasion though I didn't trust my carer enough to tell him who I was trying to telephone because, as far as I believed, he was in on it. I was becoming agitated and it was time to take action. I got out of bed and stood, without any problem at all it seemed, despite my weakened condition. I was immediately told to get back into bed and gently pushed back onto it, the longsuffering pressure mattress beneath me letting out its wheezing breaths every time I landed on it.

Just as immediately, I got back up again. Meanwhile, the imaginary Brenda had joined me by the side of the bed. I had started seeing other people on the ward who I worked with back in Wales. The imaginary Brenda was by my side supporting me just in case my legs gave way. I whispered in her ear, conspiratorially. "Ooh. That's interesting. See those two coming in?" I pointed to some staff or visitors probably. "They work for the Council." *Surely, they're not taking part in this filth?* I thought. The imaginary Brenda asked me if I worked for the Council. "What sort of a question is that?" I snapped back at her. "You know I do!" I looked at her incredulously. *There's something very wrong here,* I thought. Twenty years on and off, I've worked with her and she's acting like she knows nothing about me.

By now, a doctor had been summoned due to my bizarre behaviour. He approached me. I was still standing at the side of my bed with the imaginary Brenda. I had started to become a little challenging by this point.

"Hello Kev. I'm David. Do you remember me? I was one of the doctors who treated you when you were first admitted." As far as I was concerned, I had never seen this man before in my life and he was preventing me from going about the serious business at hand.

"No. I don't remember you. You're not particularly memorable." I said, perfunctorily and cuttingly. I proceeded to try to negotiate my way around him. He moved sideways to block me, saying that I should get back into bed. "I don't want to get back into bed. I'm fed up with being in bed!" I tried again to get around him, but he blocked me again and repeated he thought it best I get back into bed, pushing me back as he said so. I'd had enough of this now.

"Look, fuck off! Stop pushing me onto the bed. I don't want to get back into bed! I know my rights! And I know what's going on here. I think it's disgusting! I'm going to report you to your professional body." I continued. I wasn't going to reveal that I was Jim Bergerac yet or make any arrests until I knew the full extent of who was involved in the hotel porn ring. The doctor insisted yet again that I get back into bed and went to push me down onto it. No way was I going to put up with this anymore! Even though on the occasions I had got out of bed I had hardly been able to stand unaided, I somehow found the strength to attempt a sprint up the corridor. It's amazing what the power of the mind can do to overcome physical weakness at times of distress.

Miraculously, and with the Hermes-footed speed and agility of Shane Williams, the former Welsh International winger, I had jinked my way around the doctor, through a gap in the gathered staff and was heading up the corridor.

However, I hadn't got very far when I felt some considerable resistance against my continued forward momentum. I was, of course, still tethered to the bed via my catheter. The catheter bag was hooked over part of the frame of my bed to keep it up off the floor. I had been stopped in my tracks because I had run the extent of the catheter's tether. "FUCK!" I rasped at the top of my unreliable voice out of frustration at still not being able to affect escape and get on with my mission. However, I wasn't about to give up. I tried running again but the same thing happened. Thankfully, for the condition of my anatomy, the catheter bag eventually unhooked itself from my bed and I was off and running again with it and its golden contents trailing on the floor behind me.

I overheard one of the assembled carers and a nurse, both women, laughing at the spectacle, commenting that there must be easier ways for a man to enlarge his penis! I continued running up the corridor, being pursued now by staff.

As I reached the end of the corridor a lady, who I immediately decided was the manager of the hotel and therefore part of the porn ring, came out of her office to my left and asked me if I was alright. I quickly remembered that I was Jim Bergerac under cover and must stay in character as this hapless person who just happened to be caught up in the middle of all this. I smiled at her and turned my head back to look out of the window where I thought I could see the highly-manicured lawns of the hotel – there were none – in fact, if my now right-minded memory serves me correctly, there was a concrete water tower in view. I said to her, "Lovely place you have here. Sorry I'm not up to participating in the film they're making."

"That's alright my love." She had a nice kindly reassuring tone to her voice. She continued, "But we are looking for an older gentleman to jump up and down naked for us on a fluffy rug while having cream doughnuts thrown at him." *Oh well,* I thought, *if that's what it takes not to draw attention to myself, then so be it.* "Oh, I could manage that." I confirmed. "Just let me know when you need me for the shot."

The staff who had followed my progress up the corridor brought me back to my bed, after checking whether I had damaged my appendage in the pseudo World's Strongest Man contest, 'Pulling a Hospital Bed by Your Penis' round. I had caused some bleeding and they would have to keep an eye on things. Indeed, I was in and out of bed and the toilet all night. I was in agony at not being able to pass urine and sweating profusely. I was hallucinating too, believing that my ward-fellow, the guy who needed to be constantly 'tucked in' by a nurse, was my wife – her face somehow superimposed on him in the bed. That was quite frightening because I was convinced that she had come to some harm (she looked wounded and scared) during the evening and I had been powerless to prevent it.

As I said, I spent a great deal of time in the toilet

that evening and during the night. I didn't know what to do with myself. It transpired that my catheter wasn't working, and I had an infection. All this was going on while I was still convinced that I was Jim Bergerac undercover. I had been in the toilet for some time, even passing out briefly. When I came to I could hear what I thought were police sirens outside – in reality no doubt it had been an ambulance. It was all over, I thought. The boys had found me and would be making arrests now. I emerged from the toilet, exhausted from yet another sleepless night and soaked in sweat from my fever, into the corridor.

However, I had done it. I had smashed the porn ring based at the hotel. Hail the conquering hero! Hearty 'well dones' and applause greeted me as I almost crawled back across the corridor to my bed. My carer was there waiting for me. He told me that the ward doctor was doing her rounds and he had informed her of my problem passing water and that I had had an 'interesting' night. Although I was happy to see him, I still wasn't convinced that he wasn't mixed up in all of this. Anyway, the ward doctor had directed the nurse to take out my catheter for good. I had been catheterised by that point for almost three weeks. The nurse charged with its removal set about the task, not prepared in my opinion, for what was about to happen. She effected its removal painlessly enough. However, as soon as the catheter was free from my body, there was an almighty whoosh as I hosed her down with the steaming pent-up contents of my bladder. She and her uniform were soaked. Of course, having been catheterised for so long, it would be some time before I would regain control of my bladder. As such, I began emptying my bladder uncontrollably and inappropriately in relation to place and time – like the elderly incontinent character, Mrs. Emery, from Lucas and Walliams' television comedy grotesquerie, *Little Britain.*

After the nurse had finished what she needed to do and fled for the nearest locker room to change, it was lunchtime. I remember it well. I had shepherd's pie. My hands wouldn't obey me that morning, they shook too much to hold cutlery. This time though I don't believe it was from alcohol withdrawal, but more likely what I had gone through the previous evening and overnight. My carer fed me. I was not clear of the confusion yet and was still Jim Bergerac.

While my carer was feeding me, the drinks trolley came around – tea, coffee, milk, bottled water, fruit juice, squash, those sorts of things. I was feeling in a good mood, what with smashing the porn ring, and wanted to make grand gestures. As I was the first person on the ward that the guy with the trolley would come to, he asked me what I wanted before anyone else. I said that I'd like to get a drink for my friend here, gesturing to my carer, sat next to my bed. The guy serving drinks enquired what he would like. I asked for a nice cold lager for him. The poor guy was flummoxed but managed to say. "I'm sorry, we don't serve alcohol here, sir." Without further ado, I turned to my carer and said, "I'm not staying here again. The bloody place is dry!"

SIXTEEN

THE TURNING POINT AND LEAVING HOSPITAL

I think that the 'porn hotel' mission and the removal of the catheter was an important watershed in my recovery. However, it was showering for the first time in three weeks that proved to be the real turning point for me. I had already been taken off the purple liquid-goo food diet and restarted on solids. I still had the nasal-stomach feeding tube in-situ though, just in case I needed to revert to the liquid diet in the event that my oesophagus couldn't withstand solid food without starting to bleed again. However, signs were getting better by the day that this was not going to happen. Indeed, my appetite for solid food was growing steadily and had already far surpassed what it had been when I was drinking. I was also taken off oxygen as my breathing was getting stronger by the day and the pneumonia, caused by the inhalation of blood during the haemorrhages, had cleared up. I was finally able to move around and start to get my balance and gradually my leg strength back, although the latter wouldn't really return until the summer of 2016 when I started to do weight training on my legs to rebuild wasted muscle.

It was amazing but the simple act of being able to take a shower by myself proved to be such an empowering act. The first shower I had was assisted by a nurse, following a controlled bowel movement early one morning. I remember it well. Rather than use a bedpan, or just make a mess in the bed (which I had never been able to prevent), I was able, at last, to control myself for enough time to let the nurse know that I needed to take a 'Number 2'. She brought a commode over to me and helped me on to it. With the curtains pulled around my bed for privacy, I took a proper, if very loose, dump! I felt like a big boy again. Then, shock and horror, I didn't have any toilet paper to clean myself up with. I reached for the call bell and back came the nurse. She was the 'old school' no nonsense type of nurse. You could liken her a bit to Nurse Crane in *Call the Midwife*. A battleaxe with a heart of gold. She told me that I didn't need toilet paper and proceeded to wipe my bottom with a wet cloth, before telling me it was about time I had a shower.

Miraculously, no sooner had the catheter been removed following Jim Bergerac's bust of the porn hotel, then I started to recover my mental faculties. On top of hepatic encephalopathy, sleep deprivation and the parasitical feeding of paranoia and dark imagination on my confused mind, it was discovered that I had been suffering from the effects of a particularly nasty urinary tract infection. Small wonder really, the amount of abuse I had given the catheter since it had been inserted and reinserted, including my World's Strongest Man attempt at pulling a hospital bed with my penis.

However, although my faculties were returning, confusion now came from a different angle. You see, hepatic encephalopathy had caused imagined situations to become real in my mind, so as a clearing mind brought with it the capability to rationalise again, I was having to consider what had and hadn't happened.

Revisiting some of the imaginary experiences and discussing them with my wife and the Marlborough Ward staff, I was beginning to realise just how confused I had been. Not that common sense returned to everything overnight. Upon leaving hospital, and for months afterwards, I would still wonder if such and such a thing had happened.

Indeed, I might never have clarity about everything that did or didn't happen.

To be honest, finding out the truth about some things was disappointing – the experiences, situations and people involved were so much more interesting than real life. The imaginary Brenda (with or without the assistance and nether-region administrations of Nurse Rubitinski) giving me bed baths was far more intriguing than the real thing had ever been. The chap in the bed next to me had not been Ray Winstone, although I am still convinced that I had tried to electrocute him. I had not made a credited appearance in Holby City, I was not Jim Bergerac and never had been – that one was a bit of a let-down! – and I had not seen people from the Council I used to work for – what a relief!

There were many more vivid examples of paranoia, imagination and sleep deprivation twisting my confused mind. Too many to write about at length, such as attending the wedding of the daughter of an international criminal on a cruise ship without leaving my bed, eating bright orange breaded starfish and chips in a pub, and being in a cottage in the 1940s near an airfield used to launch bombing raids against 'Jerry' and hearing the noise of aircraft propellers. There were many more.

After I'd had my second shower, one of the nurses offered to cut the glue out of my hair, which had been used to attach the electroencephalogram electrodes to my head while I was still in Intensive Care. This was quickly followed by the same nurse carefully removing the nasal tube from my stomach. That was fantastic. As it was withdrawn everyone gave a round of applause.

I started wearing my own clothes, only shorts and t-shirts but nevertheless they represented a world of improvement over a hospital gown. I began taking longer strolls around the corridors to build up my strength, as this would be crucial to being considered for discharge. I would often stand and chat with renewed confidence to the nurses and carers at their station – having fun with them, as I had become genuinely fond of them all. I was moved to an ordinary bed without a pressure-relieving mattress – being told that I no longer needed one.

It was these sorts of things that were now speeding up my immediate recovery, bringing closer the day when I could finally be discharged.

I hadn't seen some of my regular carers for a couple of days. They were amazed when they saw the marked improvement in me, particularly after being to the dark places I had visited over the past three weeks. Then, one Friday morning towards the end of my stay in hospital, I finally got to meet one of the gastro-hepatology consultants who had treated me. He was Spanish, and his name was Juan – from that moment on he became known to me as 'The Juan Who Had Saved My Life'. Juan spent some time with me that morning, advising me about what had happened and what had caused it. He described what had happened as "truly scary", that I had almost been lost on more than one occasion after suffering one of the worst bleeds he had seen in the years he had been practising. As a result, he confirmed that I must never have alcohol again, as the same thing would undoubtedly happen and next time I would not be so lucky. At the end of our chat he agreed that I could go home the following Monday as I so obviously wanted (and needed) to.

EPILOGUE

THE NEVER-ENDING
PAIN OF
UNREQUITED LOVE

SEVENTEEN

AFTER HOSPITAL AND THE REALITIES OF LIFE WITHOUT 'HER'

While I was in hospital, Jan and I had received many messages of support and love. Early on, when I was in my induced coma in Intensive Care and my life was at its lowest ebb, a former colleague of mine was lighting candles for me in church. I have never been, and am still not, despite surviving this closest of shaves, a religious person in the conventional sense. By that I mean I do not subscribe to the artifice and expedience of man's various interpretations of divinity, and the pseudo-supernatural conventions of the institutions he has created and established for worship. However, it touched me, deeply, simply to know that this person cared enough to do this for me and Jan, as she believed it to be the most powerful way in which she could help us.

I left hospital on 24th November 2015. I was still extremely weak. My legs were jelly-like. I was not able to walk very far without assistance and I became fatigued very quickly. I still couldn't use my voice properly either, which continued to be a source of great frustration. Now that I had my mental capacity back to about 90%, I began to recognise and understand the yearning pain of wanting to drink. I realised that okay, I had survived the immediate crisis but the hard work of long-term survival, if it was to be, was about to begin.

Having left hospital only a month before Christmas, 'she' was the poster girl who was everywhere. There were advertisements for alcohol in all its infinite varieties. Ordinarily, Christmas had been a time for excess on all levels for me, but especially the consumption of alcohol. Christmas was the licence I required to double the company of my lover. I could enjoy drinking on two levels at the same time – the open and the clandestine.

Her presence that Christmas was heightened to an extreme for me. I could see her everywhere. It was a bit like the first Christmas after breaking up from a significant flesh and blood, emotional and physical, human lover. I felt sad that I would not be able to enjoy the festive season with her as I had before. I assumed that Christmas was going to be miserable, an intolerable and painful waste of time without her.

However, I got through that Christmas. My wife had even offered not to have alcohol in the house ever again, including at Christmas time, if it would help me steer clear of her. I wouldn't hear of that though, as I didn't want to let my mistakes limit my wife's enjoyment of life any more than I had already. Besides, it is a necessary step for the recovering alcoholic to learn to live with the presence of alcohol and not try to deny its very existence, which, of course, is impossible.

Due to the need for constant vigilance against alcohol and surveillance of those areas of my health which alcohol has damaged, it could be said that I am now consuming my life in six monthly servings, coinciding with the surveillance checks on my liver looking for hepatocellular carcinoma (hepatomas for short). These are malignant tumours which can develop in the livers of people with liver disease and cirrhosis.

My life is one of constant surveillance in several ways - constantly monitoring the triggers which might get pulled, ending up with me being reconciled with 'her'; and the ultrasound scanning of my liver and kidneys every six months, in June and December. I should also have endoscopies to monitor the development of further oesophageal varices, but I've refused to have them as the mere thought of having to endure that procedure with such regularity, let alone go through them, would encroach upon the enjoyment of my life.

As a reminder that I will never truly be out of the woods and free of her control over what is left of my life, following my routine ultrasound scan on 20th December 2017, I had a considerable scare. These scans are painless and performed by a sonographer. I was expecting this scan to find no problems, as I was in very good shape, having been working out, eating very healthily and, of course, had remained 100% abstinent from alcohol. I'd also had several ultrasound scans by this time, so knew the drill in terms of the sequence of where the sonographer would apply the transducer probe and how long they had taken previously. On this occasion, however, about halfway through the scan she seemed to be returning repeatedly to a spot on my right side between my liver and right kidney. Because of this the scan was also taking significantly longer than any of the previous ones I'd had.

Even before the sonographer had completed the scan, I was beginning to think maybe something was wrong. When she had finished and while I was getting dressed I asked, as I always do, how things were looking - joking nervously whether I was expecting twins. However, she had a serious look on her face and stated that she thought she had seen shadows on my liver in the area next to my right kidney. She said that she would email my consultant straightaway and send him the images to check over. She added that my consultant would be in touch with me, probably to initiate further tests. In the meantime, she wished me good luck and a merry Christmas...

For the next couple of weeks, I was in my own private hell. I tried not to show how scared I was, but I was 'bricking it' and my poor wife was having to share, yet again, in the tribulations I felt I was bringing to our lives. My consultant telephoned me over Christmas to ask me to come in for an MRI scan and reminded me in that conversation that I was now predisposed to developing the aforementioned tumours. I had the MRI scan a couple of days later, numbed by fear and diazepam. My consultant telephoned me immediately after the images had been analysed and confirmed that they showed nothing irregular, except for what we already knew. I didn't just breathe a sigh of relief – my legs went from under me as euphoria came over me when what seemed the heaviest of weights was lifted off my shoulders. This euphoria didn't last long though, as my mind almost immediately posed the question: *What about the next time...?*

EIGHTEEN

'DO NOT GO GENTLE...'
GO ONWARDS!

In the Prologue to this story, I spoke about the inadequacies in our society to respond to mental illness and its manifestations on the same level that it does physical diseases and incapacities. Having got through the initial trauma of what happened to me in November 2015, one of the first things that came to my newly crystal-clear mind was that I wasn't going to allow being a depressive and an alcoholic to define me.

If it comes to defining how some others see me, (people who are personally acquainted with me, but short of being true friends) that is a perception I can only try to change through gentle argument and persuasion – should I ever feel the need to. However, for those who will never be able to see me, and therefore probably all depressives and alcoholics, other than those things first, and everything else second, their attitudes probably say more about them than anything they believe is truly negative about me.

Therefore, it's their problem.

I am now very open about my alcoholism. By that I don't mean I approach people in the street and introduce myself, "Hello, I'm Kevin, I'm a recovering alcoholic." What I mean is that there are occasions that could be awkward without this openness, where there are people, or new friends, who don't know me very well, or who don't know what happened to me. For example, on being offered an alcoholic drink and declining it for a soft drink, it's not uncommon for the person doing the offering to press me to have one (because you have to drink alcohol don't you?) and I simply say that I don't drink alcohol. If they continue to press me, "What, never ever?" and I tell them "No." If they press again, "Why is that?" I say, "Because I am a recovering alcoholic." It tends to shut down the conversation for a split second, but its best to be upfront when pressed in order to avoid having to go through the game of charades if one is in a social situation with that person again.

However, for a short time after leaving hospital and returning home, the fear of being defined as a drunkard was very real. When I first started to see people again I was very worried that they would have lost any respect they might have had for me before, after I confirmed that the crisis I had just had in my life and health was acutely due to alcoholism and chronically to depression.

If some people persist in defining alcoholics by recourse to the same old tired and stereotypical trope of the 'drunkard no-hoper', I can only hope that such stale and entrenched attitudes will gradually be eroded, and eventually washed away by the long overdue rising tide of understanding; to be replaced by a growing and more healthy knowledge and opinion of depression, addiction, alcoholism and the alcoholic. I am optimistic that this will eventually happen. However, a lot rides on the implementation of the genuine intent of the Health and Social Care Act 2012 and if this successfully leads to the creation of true parity of esteem.

During the time that has passed since I left hospital, I have been evaluating what happened to me, what I have learnt from it, and still need to learn. I don't believe I've been obsessed by it all, but I suppose it is only natural to try and make sense of such a traumatic episode in one's life.

I believe that what happened to me in November 2015 was a truly galvanising, possibly you could even call it a life-affirming experience. It was certainly a positive experience – it stopped me drinking after all. Indeed, on leaving the safety of hospital, I simply had to see, understand and nurture the positives that had come from the trauma I had just experienced, and carry them forward as part of the armoury I will always need to don in my fight against her constant efforts.

Immediately, I knew that in some respects my life could, should and never would be the same again. Due to the poor state of my mental health, I knew that I could never afford to have contact with my family again.

I also knew straight away that I would never be able to return to my job. My now former employer had been very supportive of me during my times of illness, but I knew that only so much allowance could be made for me and the impact my regular and prolonged absences were having on the service. Added to that was my personal need to break with as much of the past as I could. Therefore, like my relationship with my family, my relationship with my employer of over thirty years would also have to come to an end.

However, being only forty-nine, I was far too young to retire, and certainly could not afford to do so financially. This meant that I needed to find something else to do to make a living. Therefore, I decided to work for myself, helping private residential and nursing home providers to maintain the quality of their services. This allowed me to work when I wanted to, and not throw away the skills and experience I had developed over the years. I was very kindly offered work by the owner of a care home near to where I was living at the time, and this eased me into the world of working for myself.

However, I wanted to do more than this, and so decided to write this story, and a second one, at least, on the causes of my depression, in the hope that it might be of use to others in the grip of depression and alcoholism. As the great Dylan Thomas wrote:

Though wise men at their end know dark is right,
Because their words had forked no lightning they
Do not go gentle into that good night.

I wanted to show others that they can get through this, live fully and make a positive contribution again before it's too late. I won't lie and say it's easy. It's hard! My rebirth was certainly bloodier than my birth, and I am now going through considerable growing pains again – but I'm still alive and alertly so. Yes, I still have black moments when my depression bites me, but I'm not stumbling about in a permanent numb miasma of booze-fed melancholia. I've done that, and as painful and imperfect as it will always be to some degree, I certainly prefer the clarity of my life as it is now.

Lightning Source UK Ltd.
Milton Keynes UK
UKHW020613100419
340798UK00015B/1121/P

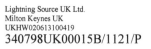

9 781789 420326